Multiple Sclerosis and
(lots of)
Vitamin D

Multiple Sclerosis and *(lots of)* Vitamin D

ANA CLAUDIA DOMENE

My Eight-Year Treatment with
The Coimbra Protocol for Autoimmune Diseases

To all those who are taking ownership of their healing process, and turning great health challenges into great personal victories.

Contents

Acknowledgments

Thank you to my husband, Robert, for his unwavering support and for our lovely partnership. Thank you so much to the members of the MS discussion groups to which I belong. You helped me with your vast experience when I had none, and continue helping me with your knowledge and friendship. A special thank you to the patients who agreed to send me their testimonies for this book. May your words reach many. And my deep, heartfelt thanks to Dr. Cicero Galli Coimbra, for having the courage to put the best interest of his patients' above any other interest, and for giving me back my life.

Disclaimer

The health information contained in this book is for educational purposes only and it is not intended as a medical manual. It represents my opinions, based on my personal experience with multiple sclerosis and the treatment with high-dose vitamin D. My intention is not to diagnose or treat any condition; rather, it is to educate and inspire you to explore a therapeutic approach that has enabled thousands of patients around the world to keep their autoimmune diseases in permanent remission. All warranties are disclaimed, without limitation, as well as liability for any damages arising from the use and/or application of the contents of this book, either directly or indirectly. The protocol discussed in this book is a medical treatment, and must always be carried out under the supervision of a qualified medical doctor.

Introduction

*"I did as much research as I could and I took
ownership of this illness, because if you don't take care
of your body, where are you going to live?"*

– Karen Duff

If you picked up this book, chances are you have been or are
in the process of being diagnosed with an autoimmune disease.
You might even be following a treatment plan and taking the
medications your doctor prescribed for your condition. But you
are still searching for a solution, because the truth is that when it
comes to autoimmune diseases, conventional medicine has failed
miserably.

For my own condition, multiple sclerosis, the conventional
options available today are powerful drugs that might or might
not affect the progression of my disease, might or might not ease
my symptoms, and would surely disrupt my life with their long
list of harsh side effects. I took one of those drugs for almost two
years, until I realized it was at best a palliative; it was far from
being a solution.

My purpose in writing this book is to give you a straight-
forward, practical look into the protocol that has become my
solution. I won't dwell on detailed explanations of what autoimmune disorders are, or talk extensively about conventional
treatment options, diet plans or stress management. There are
great resources available about each one of those subjects, and I
recommend that you research them, for it makes a difference to

be up-to-date about topics that can affect your condition. I'll talk briefly about those subjects, but only as they relate to my own experience. What I really want to share with you is the treatment I ultimately chose for myself. I want you to know how I found this treatment and what it has done for me in the eight years since my diagnosis. I want to enable you to choose it as well, if you so wish.

In 2002, a Brazilian neurologist, Dr. Cicero Galli Coimbra,[1] noticed that, in order to raise their levels of vitamin D, patients with autoimmune diseases required higher doses than the average population. That was the beginning of what is presently known as the Coimbra Protocol.

In this book, I share my experience with the Coimbra Protocol. The information expressed here is based solely on what I've learned as a patient, but it should be enough to give you an idea about this treatment plan, as well as allow your doctor a general understanding of it, should you request her assistance with the necessary medical tests. Let me reiterate: In order to follow this protocol, you must consult with a doctor who is knowledgeable in high-dose vitamin D treatment. At the end of the book, in Resources, you'll find a link to the updated list of doctors. Afterwards, your own physician can request the laboratory tests, but you must have the supervision of a doctor who understands the Coimbra Protocol, someone you can turn to whenever you have questions about your treatment progress or personal test results.

I'm from Brazil, where Dr. Coimbra practices. I am also a patient of Dr. Coimbra, though I have lived in New Mexico, USA, for the last 20 years. My own primary care physician, here in Albuquerque, has been ordering all my lab tests since I started taking high doses of vitamin D. This doctor is an MD, a conventional physician who works for a major hospital in the state; still, he has been very supportive of my choice of treatment. I believe that many doctors in this country would be just as supportive.

Presently, there are doctors in Canada, the United States, Italy, Portugal, Spain, Croatia, Argentina, Peru and Brazil prescribing the Coimbra protocol. As patients become aware of this option and request it, a growing number of doctors are becoming interested, making it available to more people with autoimmune diseases.

In chapters 4, 5, and 6, I tell my own story to give you a hands-on example of what to expect with this treatment. I talk about how often I have lab tests done, what my MRI results have shown through the years, how the diet works, etc. I try to keep it brief and to the point, because I know that what you are really looking for is an answer to the question: "Can this be a solution for me?"

In Chapter 10, there are testimonies from other patients who follow the Coimbra Protocol. During one of my trips to São Paulo, I had the privilege of personally meeting some of them; others I have known for quite some time from our Facebook groups. They are patients of relapsing-remitting multiple sclerosis, primary progressive multiple sclerosis, rheumatoid arthritis, Crohn's disease, psoriatic arthritis, and psoriasis. I'll let their words speak for themselves.

As you read through the various sections, you'll notice that this is not a book about learning how to live with a disease, nor about drastically changing your diet and lifestyle to achieve healing. This book is about a medical approach that can ease your symptoms, get you off your medications, and restore your health. It's about how powerful the right treatment can be. Sometimes it's difficult to accept that such complex disorders can have such a simple solution as taking vitamin D, so let me share this story with you.

In 1595, the world faced a serious problem with sailing ships. Sailors were dying from a silent disease, with no apparent cause. In 1601, Captain James Lancaster decided to give a teaspoon of lemon every day to part of his crew. The result was that among the sailors that took the lemon, no one died. Among the ones who did not take the lemon, the mortality rate was about 40 percent. Captain James told everyone about it, but to no avail. In 1753, James Lind, a ship's doctor, published a study comparing six different approaches to the prevention and treatment of the disease, which by then had been identified and named scurvy. In this study, he concluded: *"The most sudden and visible good effects were perceived from the use of oranges and lemons."* Still, nobody thought about implementing the use of lemons in ships. In 1865, the intake of lemons was finally recommended as a prevention for scurvy, but because doctors did not understand how lemons cured the disease, this prevention practice was soon discredited. For the next 60 years, scurvy continued killing people – despite having a known solution, with scientific research to back it up. This went on until 1932, when vitamin C was finally isolated and doctors understood that scurvy was caused by a deficiency of vitamin C, something easily solved with one teaspoon of lemon a day.

To this date, there are thousands of scientific, peer-reviewed studies showing a link between vitamin D levels and autoimmune diseases. Let's hope that it doesn't take 300 years until realistic doses of vitamin D start being recommended for prevention and treatment of these disorders.

Finally, if you are wondering whether I'm living well with multiple sclerosis these days, I can honestly say that I am, that despite being diagnosed at age 40, a fact that increased my probability of having a more aggressive disease, I barely remember I have MS.

That's why I've become so passionately determined to talk about vitamin D to all those with autoimmune conditions. In the last eight years, I've been very active in social networking, mainly in groups and forums from Brazil. Now, being on the Coimbra Protocol for so long and with such remarkable success, I believe this treatment needs to be known by patients everywhere.

Because I started taking high doses of vitamin D so early in my diagnosis, my life is vastly different from what I once feared it would be, and I hope the information you find in this book will allow you to experience the same.

Chapter 1

"Vitamin D is cholecalciferol, a hormone. Deficiencies of hormones can have catastrophic consequences."

– Dr. William Davis

Vitamin D

We've learned to think of vitamin D as a vitamin, a substance we get from our diets, like vitamin C or vitamin B12. It was named as a vitamin because it was discovered early in the last century, when scientists detected it in cod liver oil. As scientists had already identified vitamin A, some B vitamins and vitamin C, they imagined the new substance as being vitamin D. But despite its name, vitamin D isn't really a vitamin, and we can't rely on our diets to obtain it. Rather, we make vitamin D in our skin by absorbing ultraviolet light from the sun.

It took a few decades for researchers to realize that this substance is, in fact, a hormone. In 1931, the German chemist Adolf Windaus showed that vitamin D has a similar structure to steroid hormones. However, it differs from other hormones in the fact that while specific hormones target specific organs, every tissue and cell in our body has receptors for vitamin D. Today, vitamin D is considered a secosteroid hormone, a substance in a class by itself, a biochemical key that controls at least 229 of our genes and opens thousands of essential processes in our cells.

Over 25,000 of our cellular functions depend on adequate levels of vitamin D, including the role this substance plays in modulating the immune system. When the levels of vitamin D are sufficient, our cells will work properly. But when our levels are low, many of these functions will fail.

A study published by the University of Colorado in 2009[2] showed that three-quarters of teenagers and adults in the US are deficient in vitamin D. In the wake of this study, the Institute of Medicine (IOM) decided to review its recommended daily dose of 200-600 IU (International Units). However, at the end of 2010, despite the widespread deficiency of vitamin D in the country, the IOM elected to maintain its recommendation: "A recommended daily value of 600 IU was set for children ages one year and older, as well as for adolescents, pregnant and lactating women, and adults as old as 70."[3]

Meanwhile, Dr. Michael Holick, the world's leading vitamin D researcher, states: "All teenagers and adults can easily tolerate 10,000 IU of vitamin D a day without concern for toxicity."[4] Dr. John Cannell, founder of the Vitamin D Council and author of numerous peer-reviewed papers on vitamin D, agrees: "They might think it's toxic," says Dr. Cannell during an interview regarding the safety of vitamin D, "but they can't find a case in the medical literature in the history of the world that shows it is. They can't even find a case where somebody taking 10,000 IU of vitamin D a day – for no matter how many years – experienced vitamin D toxicity. Vitamin D toxicity would generally start to appear if someone was taking 50,000 IU a day for many months. Even in that case, 50,000 IU a day won't be toxic for everybody. Vitamin D toxicity has never been documented to occur at blood levels less than 200 ng/ml."[5]

For Dr. Cicero G. Coimbra, the current levels recommended by health organizations around the world are not enough to get the majority of people out of deficiency. "For a healthy person," he affirms, "I can say without a doubt that 10,000 IU a day will not pose any risk, quite the contrary. For those who suffer from any autoimmune disease, this dose will provide partial relief, but will not eliminate the problem. Higher doses can be used, provided this supplementation is done under medical supervision."[6]

Chapter 2

"Absolute certainty rarely exists when it comes to making decisions of any kind. For vitamin D, the real question is, how much evidence do we need before we act on what we already know?"

— Dr. Reinhold Vieth

Vitamin D and Autoimmune Diseases

The function of the immune system is to protect us against disease and infection. All of our cells have receptors on their membranes that allow the immune system to recognize our cells as part of our body, and in a healthy person the immune system will be able to distinguish which cells are "safe" and which are a threat, like bacteria and viruses. But when the immune system doesn't function correctly, it mistakenly identifies healthy tissue as being foreign, and attacks it. Autoimmune diseases occur when the immune system misfires and the body actually starts attacking itself. This can lead to a variety of conditions, which affect different areas of the body.

In the US, approximately fifty million people are living with an autoimmune disease, estimates the AARDA (American Autoimmune Related Diseases Association), and the prevalence of these disorders seems to be on the rise. In fact, rates are developing so rapidly that autoimmune conditions are now the third leading chronic illness in this country, right behind cardiovascular disease and cancer.

The cause of autoimmunity is not completely understood.

Bacteria, viruses, toxins, food allergies, leaky-gut, drugs, and the stress of modern life all seem to play a role in triggering an auto-immune process in someone who already has a genetic predisposition to develop such a disorder. In the past few decades, another factor that has been widely researched as a possible cause for the onset and exacerbation of autoimmune diseases is deficiency of vitamin D.

The investigation about the effects of vitamin D on the immune system started about 40 years ago, when epidemiologists decided to analyze the geographic distribution of auto-immune disorders around the globe. They found out that the incidence of autoimmunity increased in direct proportion to the distance from the equator. Locations near the equator had a low prevalence of such disorders. With time, this was linked to the major effect of solar radiation on our bodies: the production of vitamin D.

To this date, thousands of published studies have associated the deficiency of vitamin D to the most common autoimmune diseases, such as lupus, rheumatoid arthritis, psoriasis, vitiligo, multiple sclerosis, and type 1 diabetes, among others.

Let's take a look at a few examples. In 2009, a study presented at the annual meeting of the American Academy of Neurology[7] found that high doses of vitamin D dramatically cut the relapse rate in people with multiple sclerosis. Patients in the high-dose group were given escalating doses of vitamin D for six months, to a maximum of 40,000 IU daily. Then doses were gradually lowered over the next six months, averaging out to 14,000 IU daily for the year. The patients given high-dose vitamin D in the study had lower relapse rate, and their T cell activity dropped significantly, when compared to the group who took lower doses. John Hooge, MD, a multiple sclerosis specialist at the University of British Columbia in Vancouver who was not involved with the research, states: "This is an impressive study that shows that even higher doses are probably safe and more effective."[8]

In 2011, a study conducted by 209 patients of systemic lupus erythematosus with the Ohio State University Medical Center[9] found that the majority of patients included in the study had vitamin D deficiency. The authors concluded that vitamin D levels were negatively correlated with lupus disease activity. In other words, the more vitamin D in the blood, the lower the lupus disease activity, and vice versa.

In 2013, a pilot study published by Dr. Danilo Finamor and Dr. Cicero G. Coimbra assessed the effect of prolonged administration of high-dose vitamin D on the clinical course of vitiligo and psoriasis.[10] In this study, nine patients with psoriasis and 16 patients with vitiligo received 35,000 IU daily for six months in association with a low-calcium diet (avoiding dairy products and calcium-enriched foods) and hydration (minimum 2.5 L daily). The clinical condition of patients significantly improved during the treatment, with no signs of toxicity observed in any of the 25 participants, including a patient with vitiligo who reached a serum concentration of 202.2 ng/ml. The results of the trial suggest that, at least for patients with autoimmune disorders like vitiligo and psoriasis, a daily dose of 35,000 IU of vitamin D is a safe and effective therapeutic approach for reducing disease activity.

Until recently, however, no study had yet proved that low levels of vitamin D could be a direct cause of autoimmune diseases. This has changed, thanks to an important study published August 25, 2015, in *PLOS Medicine*,[11] where scientists demonstrated a genetic correlation suggesting that lack of vitamin D may be a cause of multiple sclerosis. Using a technique called

Mendelian randomization, the authors examined whether there was an association between genetically reduced vitamin D levels and susceptibility to multiple sclerosis among participants in the International Multiple Sclerosis Genetics Consortium study, which involved 14,498 people with multiple sclerosis and 24,091 healthy controls. The study concluded that a genetically lowered vitamin D level is strongly associated with increased susceptibility to multiple sclerosis. According to Dr. Benjamin Jacobs, who was not involved in the research, "This study reveals important new evidence of a link between vitamin D deficiency and multiple sclerosis. The results show that if a baby is born with genes associated with vitamin D deficiency they are twice as likely as other babies to develop MS as an adult. This could be because vitamin D deficiency causes multiple sclerosis."

Regardless of all the scientific proof that vitamin D is critical in both preventing and treating autoimmune diseases, most doctors still largely ignore the facts and insist in prescribing doses of 1,000 IU to 2,000 IU daily to patients with autoimmune conditions. Thankfully, there are always exceptions to every rule, and some doctors are paying attention to these important medical findings.

Chapter 3

"Moreover, evidence-based medicine considers controlled studies dispensable when the beneficial effects are obvious. How could we administer placebos to patients with serious illnesses simply to scientifically prove the benefits of a treatment that we already know to be effective?"

– Dr. Cicero G. Coimbra

The Coimbra Protocol

What is the Coimbra Protocol?

The Coimbra Protocol is a therapeutic approach for autoimmune diseases that relies on high doses of vitamin D to halt the misguided attacks of the immune system.

Vitamin D is the most potent immunomodulator in our body. When we have adequate levels of this substance, the essential processes in our cells will unfold properly; however, according to Dr. Coimbra, all or nearly all patients with autoimmune diseases have an increased resistance to the effects of vitamin D. This resistance may be due to genetic variants, and may also be influenced by factors such as body weight, body mass index, and age. Therefore, patients with autoimmune conditions require higher levels of vitamin D to unlock the beneficial effects of this important hormone at their cells and tissue.

How did it start?

In 2002, Dr. Coimbra noticed that the recommended doses of 200-600 IU per day were not enough to raise the levels of vitamin D in patients with multiple sclerosis. He then started using the physiological dose of 10,000 IU per day, the amount our own body produces naturally when exposed to the sun for a few minutes. With this dose, Dr. Coimbra saw a remarkable clinical improvement in the vast majority of his patients. From that point on, the doses were further increased, always supported by laboratory tests to ensure patients would not experience side effects. The results were that many of these patients found themselves completely free of the symptoms and manifestations of the disease.

During the next 10 years, Dr. Coimbra and his staff gradually modified and perfected the treatment, mostly in terms of the prescribed daily doses, which grew steadily higher. From 2012 on, the desired level of efficacy was achieved and the Coimbra Protocol became very similar to what it is today.

How is the Coimbra Protocol applied?

The Coimbra Protocol requires doses of vitamin D that range from 40,000 IU to 200,000 IU per day. Usually, the dose stays around 1,000 IU per kilogram (2.2 lbs.) of the patient's weight per day. This is only the general rule, since the dose for each patient will be adjusted along the treatment, according to the lab test results.

There are instances when patients might receive an initial higher dose for a few days at the beginning of treatment. Somebody with excessive body weight, for example, might have more resistance to vitamin D. According to Dr. Coimbra, the use of higher doses can prevent relapses during the first weeks of treatment, and this can be helpful in some cases, since vitamin D requires at least two months to reach a steady level in our blood. Vitamin D may also promote remyelination of recent MS lesions, and this is another reason for using a more aggressive initial treatment in patients with demyelinating disease who have experienced a recent relapse and might be at risk of becoming disabled. The doctor will determine if a patient should start treatment with a higher dose.

During the treatment, vitamin D levels can range from 300 – 4,000 ng/ml. This is well above the normal range listed by the laboratories, which is 30 – 100 ng/ml.

Why do patients with autoimmune diseases need such high levels of vitamin D?

Patients with autoimmune diseases require higher levels of vitamin D due to their resistance to this substance. This resistance is closely related to what are called genetic polymorphisms, small mutations in our genes which are quite common. These small mutations occur spontaneously, or they can be inherited genetically or environmentally induced – smoking, nutrition, drugs, etc.

A great number of coordinated actions involving several genes are required for our body to produce vitamin D through solar exposure. If an individual has mutations in any of the genes involved in this process, she will be resistant to the biological effect of vitamin D, and will need higher doses. This is the reason why the doses are individually determined by the doctor. A patient with a mutation in only one gene or one point of this process will be less resistant. On the other hand, a patient who has mutations at different points will have a higher resistance to the actions of vitamin D.

What is the ideal level of vitamin D?

The adequate levels of vitamin D are individual; therefore, there isn't an ideal level. The test that measures the serum (blood) level of vitamin D is called 25(OH)D3. Nevertheless, vitamin D levels are not used for dose adjustments in the Coimbra Protocol. The test used to determine if vitamin D levels are adequate is the PTH – parathyroid hormone.

Parathyroid hormone, or parathormone, is a hormone released by the parathyroid glands. Vitamin D suppresses the PTH; consequently, as vitamin D levels go up, PTH levels go down. If PTH were completely suppressed, this would mean that vitamin D would be working at its maximum biological potential. Since we cannot completely suppress the PTH, for it also has its purposes in our body, we keep PTH levels at its lowest normal limit.

At the beginning of treatment, PTH levels are measured, and then measured regularly during the treatment. If PTH is not at its minimum normal limit, vitamin D daily doses are increased until the desired PTH level is achieved. During the treatment, PTH levels are expected to go down to their lowest normal limit and stay there. When this happens, the resistance to vitamin D is overcome and the patient starts benefitting from its powerful immonodulatory effects at cellular level. It usually takes two years – about four appointments – to adjust the doses of vitamin D. After this period, the treatment consists in maintenance of the proper levels of PTH and calcium.

Can anybody follow the Coimbra Protocol?

Only the doctor can determine if a patient is a good candidate to follow the Coimbra Protocol. Certain conditions might need to be addressed before the patient can take high doses of vitamin D, such as kidney or thyroid problems, among others. There are a few diseases, like sarcoidosis, that might make the patient abnormally sensitive to vitamin D. In general, the great majority of patients will be able to follow the Coimbra Protocol, but only the doctor can evaluate your health issues before you start the treatment.

Is the Coimbra Protocol effective for patients who have had an autoimmune disease for many years?

Yes. The main purpose of high doses of vitamin D is to stop disease progression, and this can be achieved even in patients who are in more advanced stages of their disease. Vitamin D might reverse previous damage as well, but it's more effective in reversing recent damage, such as demyelinated lesions in MS that are no older than two years. Therefore, even though everybody can benefit from high doses of vitamin D, as in any medical intervention, the sooner patients start treatment, the better the results will be.

Can the Coimbra Protocol be done in conjunction with the conventional treatment?

Yes. There's no harmful interaction between high doses of vitamin D and conventional medications for autoimmune diseases. The problem with doing both treatments is that vitamin D will not be as effective, since most prescription medications for these disorders are immunosuppressants, while vitamin D is a powerful immunomodulator. Usually most patients in the Coimbra Protocol stop conventional medications as soon as they feel well enough, and confident enough, to do so.

Are there side effects?

Vitamin D promotes calcium absorption in the intestines. As a result, a possible side effect of taking high doses of vitamin D for extended periods of time is an excess of calcium in the blood (hypercalcemia) or an excess of calcium in the urine (hypercalciuria). This can be avoided with a diet free of dairy and calcium-enriched foods, and regular lab tests to make sure calcium levels are kept under control.

Vitamin D is also responsible for directing calcium to the bones. However, when taken in high doses, it can take calcium out of the bones as well. These are called, respectively, osteoblastic and osteoclastic activities. To avoid the osteoclastic activity, the loss of bones mass, it's necessary to practice a daily routine of aerobic exercises, like a 30 minute walk, for example. Aerobic exercises will induce production of calcitonin and strongly inhibit osteoclastic activity, stimulating gain of bone mass.

Patients who remain sedentary in this treatment will slowly lose bone mass. Therefore, those who cannot practice aerobic exercises might need medication with time, such as bisphosphonates, to prevent osteoporosis.

These are the possible side effects of high doses of vitamin D when taken for an extended period. They are preventable by diet and exercise.

What are the necessary laboratory tests?

Doctors will request different tests depending on the specific needs of each patient. According to Dr. Coimbra, the most important measurements in the protocol are the PTH and 24-hour urinary calcium. Other measurements usually requested are total and ionized calcium, 25(OH)D3, vitamin B12, urea and creatinine, albumin, ferritin, chrome serum, serum phosphate, and phosphaturia 24 hrs, among others.

Dr. Coimbra recommends that patients have an annual bone density scan, as well as correct any vitamin B12 deficiency.

What does the diet consist of?

The Coimbra Protocol diet is very simple. Patients need to avoid dairy as well as calcium-enriched foods, and drink at least 2.5 L of liquids a day. This amount of water helps to dilute the calcium being eliminated in the urine, preventing it from being deposited in the kidneys. A few foods that are rich in calcium might also require moderation, such as nuts.

In my personal opinion, when it comes to diet, the best way to find out if you're doing it correctly is through the lab tests. If calcium levels are normal, then your diet is fine. If it's too close to the high limit, you need to avoid more foods that are rich in calcium, such as soy (tofu, soy milk), nuts, some seeds, etc.

Calcium should not be too low, either. Sometimes patients are overzealous on their dietary restrictions and end up with low calcium in the urine. If this happens, the doctor will tell you to introduce a small amount of calcium rich foods back into your diet.

Are there other recommended supplements besides vitamin D?

According to Dr. Coimbra, vitamin D is responsible for 95 percent of the treatment success. With that said, doctors do prescribe other supplements. The list of supplements and their respective doses vary from patient to patient, but the most common ones are complex B, riboflavin, B12, omega-3, magnesium, choline, chromium picolinate.

Does the Coimbra Protocol work for everybody?

The great majority of patients go into complete remission within months of starting to take high doses of vitamin D. However, a small percentage of patients find only partial relief from their symptoms, and a few experience no improvement at all.

Here are some known factors that might compromise the results of the Coimbra Protocol.

Taking excessively hot baths, or going frequently to heated pools and hot tubs, can be detrimental to the treatment. The body might interpret the change in temperature as a fever, which will activate the immune system.

Depression, anxiety and emotional stress, when left untreated, might hinder the beneficial effects of vitamin D. All emotional issues should be addressed and treated vigorously.

The occurrence of repeated infections tend to keep the immune system in a state of constant "aggressiveness", which will limit vitamin D effectiveness. Healing infections of any nature is a must for patients in the Coimbra Protocol.

Is the Coimbra Protocol a cure?

There is currently no cure for autoimmune diseases. The Coimbra Protocol is a medical treatment that, when followed correctly, can keep these disorders in remission.

Dr. Coimbra has been asked if patients will one day be able to stop taking high doses of vitamin D, or at least take lower doses, once the disease is inactive for many years. His answer is that it might be possible, but he doesn't know. Until now, no patient has shown a desire to lower her dose of vitamin D and risk having some kind of disease activity.

As it relates to my own experience with multiple sclerosis, I see the Coimbra Protocol as the medical treatment I follow, not a cure. The difference between high doses of vitamin D and conventional medications is that vitamin D is infinitely more effective in preventing relapses and stopping disease progression, and much safer, with less significant side effects. The few side effects of this treatment are preventable, which doesn't happen with conventional treatments. No amount of diet and exercise can prevent the side effects caused by prescription medications for multiple sclerosis.

After being on the Coimbra Protocol for eight years, I still have multiple sclerosis. I will likely always have multiple sclerosis. But for me, having MS now is like having a much less scary chronic condition, like diabetes or high blood pressure. As long as I take my very effective medicine – vitamin D, the disease remains inactive.

—⁓—

I hope I was able to convey to you a general idea of how the Coimbra Protocol works, and why taking high doses of vitamin D has very different results than only supplementing with vitamin D.

It's important to remember that this treatment must always be carried out by a qualified physician. If not administered correctly, doses higher than 10,000 IU per day can cause irreversible damage to the kidneys, among other complications.

Chapter 4

"The deficiency of vitamin D is practically a pre-requisite for the development of any autoimmune disease."

– Dr. Cicero G. Coimbra

My Diagnosis

One morning, in the beginning of 2008, I woke up with a light tingling in my feet. I thought maybe I had exercised too much the day before and was having some kind of reaction. But as the day went on the tingling slowly climbed up my legs, and by the time I left work I was feeling it in my whole body, from the neck down.

That was how my story with multiple sclerosis started. I spent the next few weeks going through test after test, seeing a variety of specialists who ordered CT scans, blood work, MRIs and finally a spinal tap. During that period, my symptoms got much worse. By the time I finally heard the words multiple sclerosis, I was experiencing tingling and numbness throughout different parts of my body, I had lost control of my right arm, I had developed a weakness in my left leg, and I felt such intense fatigue that even standing up for a few minutes left me exhausted.

When the spinal tap results came back positive for oligoclonal bands – a protein present in the spinal fluid – I was diagnosed with multiple sclerosis. This might sound strange, but my first reaction was relief. I knew there was something very wrong with me, and a few possibilities being investigated by the doctors were even scarier than multiple sclerosis. Besides, during the previous weeks, I had done a fair amount of research on some of the diseases that could be causing my problems. In my readings, I had gotten the impression that certain autoimmune diseases seemed to become more manageable when patients followed specific diets, exercised regularly, and kept a healthy lifestyle. These things made sense to me; I knew I could change my lifestyle if I needed to. So, when the neurologist said I had multiple sclerosis, I felt somewhat relieved.

However, my relief was short lived because the doctor immediately went on to explain the treatment. I had four options, all of them injectable medications. Three were in a class of drugs called interferons, and the other was an immunomodulator called copaxone. Apparently, they all had similar efficacy, but copaxone had fewer side effects. The doctor said that in my case she recommended copaxone.

How effective was copaxone? It would prevent about 30 percent of relapses, and it might or might not slow down the progression of the disease. That did not seem very effective to me, but since the doctor had said that the side effects were not as bad, I thought there would be no harm in taking it. When I got home, I looked up the side effects: chest pain, severe rash or skin irritation, dizziness, sweating, trouble breathing, pounding heartbeats, fluttering in the chest, weakness, back pain, swelling in hands or feet, fever, chills, body aches, flu symptoms, double vision, among many others.

At the time, I was really trying to be positive, but I started to wonder how that drug could benefit me; it seemed to have so many more cons than pros. Too many side effects – long and short term – for too little benefits. Still, back then I didn't have the knowledge nor the confidence to refuse conventional treatment. As far as I knew, that was my best option.

I started taking copaxone, but intuitively, I believed there had to be a better way. In my search for alternative treatments, I found many testimonies of patients that had chosen different routes, usually diets and supplementation of vitamins. These approaches were meant to work with the body's natural healing ability instead of hindering it with drugs. I was not sure if it would be enough to stop multiple sclerosis completely, but I was determined to try.

One of the websites that helped me a great deal was Ashton Embry's MS charity website, Direct MS. I decided to start following the diet recommended by them, the Best Bet Diet, which suggested avoiding foods such as dairy, beans, soy, sugar, gluten, among others, and taking a variety of supplements. The Direct MS website was also full of scientific references, and one area of research that grabbed my attention immediately was the possible link between vitamin D and multiple sclerosis. In a few weeks, I read dozens of studies on the subject. Vitamin D was one of the supplements recommended by the Best Bet Diet, and I started taking the suggested dose of 5,000 IU a day.

In some MS forums, I met patients that had upped their dose to 10,000 IU a day and felt great improvement in their symptoms. I was wondering if I should do the same, but as often happens in life, when you're on the right track things just fall into place. One late afternoon, a very dear friend from Brazil, Cristiane, called to ask how I was doing in my search for a diagnosis. She knew I had been unwell but didn't know yet I had multiple sclerosis. I told her that I had already found out what was wrong with me, that she shouldn't worry, it sounded serious but nowadays there were many new and excellent treatments—

"Just tell me what it is, Ana." She was never the patient type.

"Multiple sclerosis."

"Multiple sclerosis?"

"Yes."

"Ah… don't worry, you'll be completely fine."

She was so nonchalant that I was sure she was thinking of a different illness, but I agreed. "Yes, Cris. There are many new treatments—"

"No, no, no. Do you know who else has multiple sclerosis? Isabel." Isabel was a mutual friend of ours. I had no idea she had MS. "Isabel has had MS for years. She takes some vitamins and she is doing great."

Since I was taking vitamins and particularly interested in vitamin D, I was immediately curious. I told her I was following a diet that also prescribed vitamins.

"This is different, Ana. There is a doctor in São Paulo that treats MS with vitamins, but not in regular doses. High doses. Isabel has been his patient for many years. She says since she started this treatment, she has forgotten she has MS."

"That sounds wonderful, Cris. I'll talk to Isabel."

"Talk to her and come to Brazil. And don't worry about this disease anymore; soon you'll be completely fine."

Chapter 5

"When we started with vitamin D and found out that it was effective, we made a life choice. We left academia behind – this thing of drugs here, drugs there, launches of drugs, testing of new drugs, allegedly satisfactory successes. We put it all aside and thought only of the interest of the patient who was there, at our office, in that moment."

– Dr. Cicero G. Coimbra

The Treatment

I talked to Isabel in August of 2008. She had been diagnosed with MS four years earlier, and for six months she had taken avonex, one of the interferons prescribed for multiple sclerosis. The injections gave her severe side effects, and she felt she was slowly losing her quality of life. After six months of being on avonex, her doctor requested MRIs and she found out she had developed new lesions on her brain. She felt lost, and she did not know if it was worth it to keep taking the medication and enduring the side effects, when it didn't seem to be working. It was then that her pharmacist told her about Dr. Cicero Coimbra and his treatment with high doses of vitamin D. She liked what she heard and scheduled an appointment with him. She started feeling better almost immediately. Her fatigue was gone after a couple of months, other symptoms from the disease soon followed. She stopped taking avonex, and felt she had gotten her life back. After taking vitamin D for one year, she repeated her MRIs, which showed no disease activity and no new lesions. Almost four years later, nothing had changed. She felt great.

It's now been 12 years since Isabel started her treatment with high doses of vitamin D. To this day, she has not had another flare up, has not experienced any side effect from vitamin D, and is completely healthy. Today Isabel is 45 years old, an age in which MS tends to get more aggressive, especially if you've had it for 12 years. Nevertheless, she says she feels absolutely nothing related to the disease.

When I talked to Isabel, back in 2008, she told me she would see Dr. Coimbra in a couple of weeks and that she would mention my case to him. I was not sure when I would be able to go to Brazil for an appointment, but I asked her to let him know I was already taking 5,000 IU a day. Isabel told me she was taking 25,000 IU daily.

Isabel talked to Dr. Coimbra about me, and he said that as long as I found a doctor that would order the necessary lab tests, I could start taking 15,000 IU daily. This is a very safe dose, since our own body produces this amount if we stay in the sun for about 20 minutes. Still, as a precaution, he said I should avoid dairy and calcium-enriched foods.

I was elated. I've always considered myself a very intuitive person, and from the early days of my diagnosis, nothing had grabbed my interest as much as vitamin D. I was hopeful that the higher dose would alleviate my symptoms, which were still very intense, even after three months of following the Best Bet Diet and taking copaxone.

In truth, my symptoms had gotten so much worse that, thinking back, I realize I probably had a second flare up in the midst of getting the diagnosis and starting treatment. Reading about MS, I found out that I checked all the marks for factors that indicate a higher risk of a more severe, aggressive disease. I was 40 years old, my initial symptoms had affected more than one area of my body, and my first flare up affected motor control. But I didn't need to read about MS to know that mine was aggressive, and I was desperate to find something that could at least calm it down. Finding a doctor that was already prescribing vitamin D in high doses made me believe that maybe my instincts had been right, and that I had found the solution I was searching for.

I went to see my primary care physician and told him about my plans to up my dose to 15,000 IU per day. I had already decided that if he didn't agree to order my tests I would look for a naturopath or functional medicine doctor, who are usually more open to unconventional therapies. Despite my apprehension, he agreed promptly. He seemed to be very knowledgeable about vitamin D, and didn't appear concerned about my dose being too high. As long as the tests showed no side effects, he would help me with the treatment. Now I was truly elated.

I have to say that this doctor has my deepest respect and gratitude. He still orders all the necessary lab tests every six months, and in each of my appointments, he rejoices in my continuing good health. The world needs more doctors like him, open to listening to their patients, and open to new ways of dealing with diseases, mainly the ones that have no effective treatment in conventional medicine.

I left his clinic, went home, and started my new daily dose of 15,000 IU. I also kept on taking copaxone and following the Best Bet Diet.

—◊—

Vitamin D did not let me down. The improvements came slowly, but within the first few weeks I could tell that the symptoms were not getting any worse. After about three or four months, my extreme fatigue started to ease, and I could do things around the house without feeling completely drained.

After six months, I had my first lab tests done and everything came back normal. The only result out of the normal range was 25(OH)D3, which was at 130 ng/ml. The top limit is set at 100 ng/ml. But that result was expected because I knew that following the Coimbra Protocol, my vitamin D levels could go much higher than that.

It was after seven months that the changes really kicked in. My right arm was not so clumsy, I was able to tie a shoelace and hold a glass of water without spilling it, my leg didn't feel as weak as before, and the tingling in my legs disappeared, followed by the tingling in my torso and arms. It took seven months for the improvements to start, but once they did, the progress was very fast. Nine months after having increased my dose, I felt I was almost back to normal. The only reminder I had of MS was a constant tingling on my right hand and left fingers, which has never disappeared and is with me to this day. My improvements felt remarkable. I was ecstatic and anxious to see what the MRIs would show.

———

During those months, I was also trying to deal with severe anxiety, which might have been caused physically, by the illness itself, or emotionally, by the stress of the health situation I was living in. My primary care prescribed an antidepressant but I didn't feel it was enough, so I decided to look for a therapist and found a wonderful, supportive psychoanalyst whom I saw once a week for the following two years.

This not only helped me with anxiety, but it was one of the best decisions of my life. I gained self-knowledge, and I grew and learned and changed. I became less scared of the disease, and I believe that was an important step towards healing.

Another thing that helped me in those first months was acupuncture. It eased some of my symptoms and helped with my sleep, which brought a great improvement for my health in general. I also made an effort to start exercising again, even if only for a few minutes a day. I was determined to do everything in my power to become physically and emotionally healthier.

—⁓—

When I completed one year of treatment with vitamin D, I went back to my neurologist and she ordered spinal cord and brain MRIs. She was not as enthusiastic as my primary care had been about my experiment with vitamin D, but she told me that as long as I stayed on copaxone and my clinical tests were fine, she would not tell me to stop it. I remember one occasion when she offered to request some of the necessary tests for the Coimbra Protocol, which sent the whole clinic into an uproar, for nobody knew how to request the calciuria 24 hrs test. The code for it was not in their computers, and for a while nurses and doctors got totally caught up in figuring out how to get it. It took about 20 minutes, but in the end I left with the order for my test. I know I have been extremely lucky in my conventional doctors, and I do make a point of thanking them every time we meet.

In December of 2009 I did my first MRIs after my diagnosis. I had been on high doses of vitamin D for about 16 months. My neurologist gave me the good news. I had no disease activity at all. My brain MRI showed five or six lesions, the same as the previous one. In my prior cervical MRI, I had had two lesions. A big one between C2 and C3, which measured 1.6 cm in length, and a smaller one in C4. The big one was still there, unchanged, but the smaller one had completely disappeared. I was ecstatic. I hugged my doctor. On her wall, I noticed a scientific article I had not seen in my previous visits, a recent study about vitamin D and multiple sclerosis. I left her office in the mood for a big celebration.

So, by the end of 2009 things were going well. My symptoms were much improved, the MRIs brought excellent news, I was doing psychoanalysis and acupuncture, and I was exercising again. I had also joined two online groups where members were mostly patients of Dr. Coimbra. With them, I was learning a lot about the treatment. In those groups, I found dozens upon dozens of encouraging stories, including cases where patients had arrived at Dr. Coimbra's clinic very ill, many of them after battling the disease for long years, and some for whom the medications no longer had any effect. They recovered, they felt better, and for most of them, the disease stopped progressing.

I noticed that those patients were taking between 20,000 IU and 40,000 IU daily. Since I had just done my second round of lab tests and again everything was fine, with calcium levels in the normal range, and since I had already scheduled my first appointment with Dr. Coimbra and would be seeing him in six months, I decided to increase my dose to 20,000 IU daily.

I was starting to believe that multiple sclerosis – my chronic, incurable, progressive disease – might just be something that could be beaten.

—◦◦◦—

In the beginning of 2010 I was feeling so good that I decided to ease up on the strict Best Bet Diet. I slowly introduced beans and legumes back, and occasionally I even had gluten. Since I didn't feel any worse, I resumed the eating habits I had before MS, except I still avoided all dairy products and calcium-enriched foods.

In June of 2010 I had my third round of tests done; I would be taking the results to my appointment with Dr. Coimbra the following month. In July, I headed to my long-awaited summer vacation in Brazil, anxious to see all my family and friends, as well as to meet the doctor that was changing my life.

My appointment with Dr. Coimbra lasted three hours. I have come to greatly admire this doctor for his professional brilliance and for being such a wonderful human being. I have met very few people so dedicated to others as Dr. Coimbra is dedicated to the well-being of his patients. During my appointment, he made sure he explained in detail why vitamin D was making me feel better and why it was so effective in treating autoimmune disorders. He asked questions, addressed all my doubts, and determined that I was doing everything right in terms of the diet and the lab tests. He told me I should raise my dose to 25,000 IU per day.

I left his clinic quite confident I had found a treatment that would keep me healthy for many years to come.

—◌◌◌—

Back in the US, after a great vacation on the beautiful beaches of my home country, I started taking 25,000 IU daily. I continued to feel good for a few months, until I started experiencing my first side effects from copaxone. During a visit to my primary care, he noticed that my blood pressure was a little high. I mentioned to him that occasionally I experienced a fluttering feeling in my chest, just for a couple of seconds. He ordered an EKG, which came back normal. We decided to keep monitoring the blood pressure, which stayed high. The episodes of heart palpitation became more noticeable, and soon I started feeling tightness in my chest. I thought my anxiety problem was coming back, even though I couldn't figure out why, since I was in a good place in my life. I went back to the doctor's office to ask if maybe I should take the antidepressant again. (I had already stopped it.) I mentioned to him that I didn't really feel anxious or troubled; my mind felt calm, but there was this constant tightness in my chest. He looked at my chart for a while and then turned to the computer. After a few minutes, he found what he was looking for. It was the list of side effects from copaxone; he pointed to the cardiac side effects. They were high blood pressure, heart palpitation, and chest tightness. He told me I should talk to my neurologist about stopping it. I called her office and quit copaxone that same day. The chest tightness was gone in a couple of weeks, the blood pressure took about a year to get completely back to normal, and the fluttering feeling started to happen less often; once a week, then once every two weeks, then once every few months, until it disappeared.

My biggest surprise, however, was that very soon after quitting the medication, the last of my fatigue was gone. I had been on the Coimbra Protocol for about two years and still had a light fatigue, but a few weeks without copaxone and I was back full force at the gym, lifting as much weight as I did before the diagnosis, feeling strong and full of energy.

I was done with conventional drugs for MS.

—∿∿—

In the beginning of 2011, I redid my MRIs. By then I had been on the Coimbra Protocol for two and a half years. There was no significant change in either the brain or cervical MRIs. My lab tests were also excellent. I could honestly say that the only reason I remembered having MS was the work I was doing on social networks, describing my experience with vitamin D to everyone who was interested.

This was also the year when I started investigating paleo diets for multiple sclerosis, and found Dr. Terry Wahls' recovery story on the net.[12] Before MS, I had been a vegetarian for more than a decade. Because of the Best Bet Diet, I was eating fish and seafood again. Reading about paleo diets, I started wondering if I should go back to eating red meat and chicken as well, but little did I know that before I could decide, my body would decide for me. I'll talk more about the end of my vegetarianism in the next chapter.

Before 2011 was over, I had a health problem that was not directly related to multiple sclerosis and that forced me to rethink my diet. I believe that my experience can be helpful to many people, mainly the ones with autoimmune diseases, so I'll share it with you in the next chapter.

In 2012, I became a little lax with my dairy restriction. I think I grew too confident with my continuous normal test results in almost four years of treatment, and started having a slice of pizza too many. The consequences were that in my next round of tests my ionized calcium came back at the maximum normal limit, at 1.4 mmol/L. Still normal but at the limit. My total calcium and calciuria were within the normal range. I immediately cut back on my dairy intake and repeated the test three weeks later; this time the results were what they should be, 1.32 mmol/L. Lesson learned.

All through 2012, I continued to feel well, with no manifestations from MS except the occasional tingling on my hands and arms, which seemed to get worse with exercise or heat exposure. With the years, I have grown used to this symptom; it comes and goes without ever leaving a mark on the imaging tests. It's likely an exacerbation of old symptoms, a result of the damage caused in my spinal cord by the big lesion between C2 and C3.

This was also the year when the doses prescribed in the Coimbra Protocol were increased. Because I followed the online discussion groups, I noticed that new patients were being prescribed higher doses, and old patients going back for returns usually had their dose increased. Instead of ranging from 20,000 IU to 40,000 IU, the doses now were starting at 40,000 IU and could go much higher than that.

Up to then, the patients took doses that kept their PTH levels around 20 pg/ml. But after careful observation of patients for 10 years, Dr. Coimbra noticed that the ideal individual dose of vitamin D should bring the PTH to its minimum normal level. That's when resistance to vitamin D is overcome and this hormone can function at its best potential at cellular level, as the most potent immunomodulator our body produces.

―――

At the laboratory where I do my tests, the range listed for PTH is 11 – 80 pg/ml. In the beginning of 2013, I sent an email to Dr. Coimbra letting him know that in my latest tests my PTH level was 23 pg/ml. After reviewing my latest lab work, he decided to raise my daily dose from 25,000 IU to 50,000 IU. My next tests, done after six months, showed that PTH had gone down to 18 pg/ml. It was still not all the way down to the minimum, so my vitamin D dose could be further increased. But I was feeling fine and I knew Dr. Coimbra was extremely busy; therefore I decided not to contact him again and kept on taking 50,000 IU daily.

In October of 2013, I again had MRIs done. I now had been on the Coimbra Protocol for more than five years. The MRI results were the same. No significant changes, no new lesions, no enhancement with contrast, and no disease activity. At that appointment, my neurologist told me that based on my MRIs, she would not recommend that I try any other conventional medication for MS at that moment, and that I should keep on doing exactly what I was doing. Suddenly, going in for MRIs was not so scary anymore; every time I left my doctor's office, I had a reason for celebration.

The following year, 2014, was excellent. I scheduled an appointment with Dr. Coimbra for July, during my summer vacation, but had to cancel it because the World Cup made it impossible to get tickets inside Brazil during that month. Since I had no major health concerns and all my test results were again in the normal range, I decided to postpone the appointment for another year.

—◊◊◊—

It was now the first quarter of 2015, and I had been on the Coimbra Protocol for almost seven years. A bone density test showed I had osteopenia, which meant my bone density was lower than normal peak density but not low enough to be classified as osteoporosis. Besides the high doses of vitamin D, another factor that may have contributed to my bone loss was my age. I was 47 and in perimenopause. It was very mild, but it made me realize that if I wanted to avoid medications for osteoporosis, I needed to get serious about cardio exercises. At that time, my cardio routine consisted of 20 minutes to warm up before weights, and only about three times a week. I increased it to 30 – 45 mins, at least five times a week.

By then I was determined to have my second appointment with Dr. Coimbra. It had been five years since my first and only appointment! I scheduled it for the first week of July. In preparation for it, I again repeated all the blood and urine work, which came back with excellent results, and went to see my neurologist so she could request a new set of MRIs.

This time the MRIs brought even better news than usual. While there was no significant changes in the brain MRI, there was a small change in my cervical MRI. My lesion, between C2 and C3, had shrunk 2 mm in size! It had gone down from 1.6 cm to 1.4 cm, what meant that I gained spinal volume after many years of unchanged MRIs. I had assumed that the lesion was already a scar and wouldn't change anymore, so that was a great surprise.

What exactly had happened in the last two years that could account for my lesion suddenly starting remyelinating? What happened was that in 2013, the year I had done my previous MRIs, my vitamin D dose had jumped from 25,000 IU do 50,000 IU per day. I have no doubt that achieving the correct dose and the correct levels for me, allowed vitamin D to become much more effective in my organism. I won't be surprised if my lesions keep on remyelinating.

Before doing this round of MRIs I was somewhat worried because I had been feeling more tingling than usual in my hands and arms. When the results showed I had no disease activity (only good activity!), my neurologist tried to assure me that what I felt were exacerbations of my symptoms. Still, she requested an electromyogram to investigate it further. To my surprise, the electromyogram detect a mild case of carpal tunnel, as well as ulnar tunnel, on both wrists and elbows. This could account for some of the tingling I sometimes experienced.

Discovering I had carpal and ulnar tunnel syndromes made me realize how important it is to keep in mind that not all our problems are a consequence of our autoimmune condition. We can have a number of health issues not related to our specific disease, and sometimes they go undiagnosed because we assume we already know what is causing them. Diagnosing these secondary issues can make a big difference in our health in general, and can also make our life a lot easier. By paying attention to the position of my hands and elbows, I was able to get rid of some of the tingling I was experiencing.

Going back to my latest MRIs, the shrinking of my lesion was not the only good news I got that day. For the first time the results came back with an analysis for loss of grey matter. The knowledge that patients with multiple sclerosis lose grey matter is recent. This means that, besides losing the myelin shield, patients with MS also lose neurons and the connections between them more rapidly than the rest of the population, which causes a shrinkage of the brain, or brain atrophy. This can account for the progression of cognitive and physical disabilities, even if no new lesions are detected.

A comparison of all my MRIs showed a small loss of grey matter in the first year after my diagnosis, but no loss whatsoever in the last six years. Again, the loss happened during the period when I was not yet taking vitamin D or was taking a low dose.

Once I started the Coimbra Protocol, my neurons remained intact. Coincidentally, as I write this chapter, the first study that shows that vitamin D status is positively associated with grey matter volume in patients with multiple sclerosis has just been released. The study,[13] published in the *European Journal of Neurology*, found that each 10 ng/ml increase in vitamin D levels is associated with a 7.8 ml rise in grey matter volume.

After seven years, I had no brain atrophy, no disease activity, my big cervical lesion was getting smaller, and I was free of the numerous health problems caused by conventional medications. I felt happy and optimistic. Yes, I was treading a good path, indeed.

———~~~———

I gathered all my tests and headed to Brazil and my second appointment with Dr. Coimbra. Throughout the years, we had been in contact, but it felt good to see him again, ask questions and have him look at my latest results. I had even done an ultrasound of my kidneys and urinary tract, just to make sure there were no signs of kidney stones, which there weren't. Dr. Coimbra was very pleased with my test results; however, he noticed that even with the increased dose of 50,000 IU daily, my PTH was still 18 pg/ml. He said he would feel more comfortable, and that I would be truly protected from disease activity, only when the PTH was around 11pg/ml, the minimum normal level listed by my lab.

When I told him that sometimes the tingling in my arms and hands felt more intense, he said it was possible that those symptoms were not only an exacerbation of old symptoms or caused by the carpal and ulnar syndromes. It could be that I was still experiencing subtle activity from MS, which was happening because during the seven years of treatment I had not reached my ideal dose. The activity was not enough to be detected by the MRIs, but in the long run it could cause some damage.

If it was disease activity, he wanted to know what else could be causing it, besides my vitamin D levels. He asked a few questions. Was I depressed or constantly stressed out? Did I have frequent infections? Did I take very hot showers often? The answer to the first two questions was no; to the last question was yes. I used to take two long, very hot showers a day. Besides, I used to soak in hot tubs whenever I got the chance. Dr. Coimbra recommended that I changed those habits. According to him, this is a common problem among patients who take high doses of vitamin D, because most of us don't have any heat intolerance. Therefore, we usually expose ourselves to heat more often than other MS patients do. But even though we don't feel lethargic or tired by doing so, the abrupt change in temperature can be interpreted by our body as a fever and activate the immune system. If this happens constantly, besides the exacerbation of old symptoms, too much heat exposure can promote disease activity. With time, this can bring about new symptoms, even if they are mild ones. Dr. Coimbra was not sure if I was having disease activity, but to be safe he decided to increase my daily dose to 60,000 IU and recommended that I avoid exposing myself to heat from then on.

My appointment again lasted three hours, during which he patiently answered the long list of questions I had taken with me. In the end, I left with all the answers I needed, and more certain than ever that I had found "the" treatment for MS.

After leaving Dr. Coimbra's clinic, I had a very special night in São Paulo. I went out for dinner with dozens of other patients who were following the Coimbra Protocol. Many of them I had known for many years from social media, and some of them were fellow administrators of groups we facilitate on Facebook. That night I got to personally meet patients who had been on the protocol for 13 years, 10 years, eight years, without any manifestations of the disease. That whole day was a treat to me.

—⚬—

Back in the US, I increased my daily dose to 60,000 IU, and six months later my PTH levels were finally, for the first time since I started the treatment, at 11pg/ml, the minimum normal level. As usual, all my other lab results were within the normal range. I said goodbye to my delicious hot showers. Also, when I did my cardio exercises, my body temperature increased a lot, so I bought a small USB fan and started taking it with me to the gym. I use it at the elliptical and the treadmill, and it helps to keep me cooler when I exercise. A wet towel around the shoulders is also a good idea.

Two months after increasing the vitamin D and stopping the hot showers, the tingling episodes started to become rarer. I don't know if they were some kind of disease activity or just an exacerbation of old symptoms; either way, following Dr. Coimbra's recommendations has eased the problem. Now, I experience the tingling very occasionally, mostly when I push myself too hard at the gym. I have no other symptoms or problems with MS.

So far, this is my experience with high doses of vitamin D. I intend to update this book from time to time, as I get new test results. In a few months, I'll repeat the bone density test. My hope is that I can stay away from medications and reverse the bone loss exclusively with exercises. As for MRIs, unless I experience new symptoms, I do not intend to have them done for a few years. I believe it's time to give my brain a rest from all that contrast. I'm extremely satisfied with my treatment, and my plans for now are to follow the advice of my neurologist here in the US. I'll keep doing exactly what I'm doing.

Chapter 6

"Whenever a doctor cannot do good,
he must be kept from doing harm."

– Hippocrates

Why Stomach Acid Is Good for You

The title of this chapter is the title of a book by Dr. Jonathan Wright that I can't recommend enough.[14] If you have an autoimmune disease, then you are likely to have some kind of digestive issue, even if you don't know it yet. Dr. Wright provides wonderful information about healing many of these serious potential problems and gives great insight into how they might trigger autoimmune conditions.

The experience I'll talk about in this chapter was the only health issue I've had during the eight years since my MS diagnosis. I want to share this with you because it relates to a problem many patients with autoimmune disorders might have to some degree, often without realizing. I'm also sharing it so I can stress the point of how important it is to be well informed about our health issues, to look for second and third opinions, and to think outside the box when we don't feel we are being helped by conventional medicine. The problem I had was not really serious, until I started seeing gastroenterologists and following the treatment they prescribed. It was only then that I became ill. Very, very ill.

A few years before my multiple sclerosis diagnosis, I started experiencing some minor digestive discomfort. It was nothing that concerned me, but in 2011 it started to get more bothersome. I felt sluggish after my meals, I often had episodes of diarrhea or constipation, and I started suffering from acid reflux. I decided it was time to see a specialist.

In the two months it took to get the appointment with a gastroenterologist, my acid reflux became a constant bitter taste on my mouth. I didn't experience heartburn, the more common type of reflux, as I had LPR – laryngopharyngeal reflux. In LPR, the stomach acid backs up into the throat (pharynx) or voice box (larynx), or even into the back of the nasal airway, and it can cause inflammation in areas that are not protected against gastric acid.

When I got to the doctor, I mentioned to her that the bitter taste on my mouth was always there, as well as a feeling of a lump in my throat. It didn't make a difference if I ate or not, if I was standing up or lying down, or even if I took over-the-counter antacids. The doctor requested some tests and gave me a prescription for omeprazole, a proton pump inhibitor that blocks the enzyme responsible for producing gastric acid.

As soon as I started taking omeprazole, things got worse. This was around Christmas time and my husband and I had to cancel our plans for the holidays because by then, besides the constant reflux, I was having difficulty eating. Even when I was hungry, I would feel full with very little food.

I started doing what I had already learned to do so well, research my symptoms on my own. I found a number of online forums where people talked about symptoms very similar to mine, and many of them had a condition called hypochlorhydria, or low stomach acid. This is a known medical condition, catalogued in the medical literature; however, conventional doctors mostly ignore it, insisting that gastric acid is of little value for our health, and that we may not even need it for digestion. Probably that is why it's so easy for them to prescribe acid suppressors at any signs of digestive discomfort. In most conventional hospitals, there is not even a diagnostic test for hypochlorhydria.

In my next visit, I asked the gastroenterologist about the possibility of my problem being low stomach acid. She looked at me as if she did not understand my question. She said she would schedule an endoscopy and would test my pH, the level of acidity in my stomach, but that there was no such thing as measuring the actual quantity of acid in my stomach. I explained to her that before I started taking omeprazole I had no difficulty eating; it was only after I started taking the acid blocker that I felt bloated when I tried to eat. I was wondering if maybe I was having trouble eating because my stomach had no acid to digest the food. Besides, omeprazole didn't seem to be helping with the reflux, the bitter taste on my mouth was still there. A little weaker, but still there. Her answer was that we had to keep looking for what was wrong, and that the medication was not preventing me from eating, since the stomach was able to digest food even with a very small amount of acid. She changed my prescription to Pepcid, another type of acid blocker. I started taking 80 mg a day, the maximum dose allowed.

A month after my first appointment with this doctor I had lost 12 pounds. By then, my difficulty in eating was such that I would bake a potato in the morning, leave it on the kitchen counter, and try to finish it before I went to bed at night. I took leave from work; I had to lay down constantly to rest.

I needed a second opinion, so I scheduled an appointment with the director of gastroenterology in one of the three main hospitals in New Mexico. I got to his office carrying my medical records, which by then had dozens of pages. I had had a colo-noscopy, endoscopy, numerous lab tests, adrenal glands test, abdominal ultrasound, thyroid ultrasound, celiac disease tests, and abdominal CT scan. Everything was normal, including the pH level in my stomach.

I was starting to have flash backs from my MS diagnosis, when tests kept coming back normal and I was feeling worse with each passing day. My anxiety attacks came back full force; I was not only afraid of my digestive issues but also of having a MS flare up in the midst of the stressful situation I was experiencing.

The new gastroenterologist ordered more tests, this time a gastric emptying study, esophageal manometry, esophageal pH, among others. I again asked about the possibility of my problem being low stomach acid, and he gave me the same answer I got from the previous doctor. I asked if I should try stopping Pepcid for a while to see if I could at least have less trouble eating. He told me that it would be best to wait for the tests' results to see if we could figure out what was causing all my symptoms, and that I should take the medication to keep the acid away from my throat and mouth. He told me that sometimes it took many weeks until the medication was fully effective, and instructed me to start having only liquid foods.

I was very dissatisfied with how my case was being handled. So far, the treatment was making me worse, not better. I wanted to quit the acid blockers and try taking acid supplements instead, but my throat and mouth were so inflamed that I didn't feel con-fident about changing treatments without a doctor's instruction. I was scared of trying it and making the whole ordeal worse.

By then, I had found out that in the US, it's mostly natu-ropathic and functional medicine doctors who treat reflux with acid supplements, and there's only a handful of clinics in the whole country that perform the Heidelberg test, which is considered the most accurate test for checking stomach acid levels. The nearest one to Albuquerque was in Scottsdale, AZ.

The results for the gastric emptying study came back. I had delayed gastric emptying. The doctor said I probably had gastroparesis, a disorder in which the movement of the muscles (motility) in the stomach is compromised, usually due to nerve damage. He suggested that it might have been caused by my multiple sclerosis. I was terrified. I called Dr. Coimbra immediately. He assured me that my digestive problems had nothing to do with multiple sclerosis, and openly suggested I look for a different gastroenterologist. He also told me to get MRIs done, just so I would be assured that MS was not affecting my internal organs. I went to see my neurologist and to my relief she was in complete agreement with Dr. Coimbra; in fact, she was very upset with the gastroenterologist's suggestion that multiple sclerosis might be affecting my stomach. Nevertheless, she ordered MRIs of my entire nervous system. The MRIs came back unchanged, no MS activity at all. I was relieved but not in the mood to celebrate.

Even though the MRIs were fine, I was very concerned about multiple sclerosis, because I had stopped taking my supplements, including vitamin D. My stomach would not accept the oil in the capsules, and I was no longer able to drink the 2.5 L of water required by the treatment. Without vitamin D and with the physical and emotional turmoil I was experiencing, I believed that it was only a matter of time until I had a relapse.

I went back to the gastroenterologist with the information that my MRIs didn't show any MS activity. He told me I might have idiopathic gastroparesis, meaning the problem had an unknown cause. I asked him if there was a possibility that my problem, from the beginning, had been hypochlorhydria, a known medical condition, and that the huge amount of acid suppressants I had been on was impairing my digestion. He insisted that would be very unlikely. He wanted me to redo the gastric emptying study, and a series of other tests. I let him place the order for more tests, but I was no longer paying attention to what he was saying. I had had enough. I left his office and called the clinic of Dr. Samuel Walters, in Scottsdale, to schedule the Heidelberg test.

—∕v∖—

I wanted to see Dr. Walters immediately, but was told I needed to stop taking the acid blocker for at least five days prior to the test. I went the following week. Since I was going to Scottsdale, I also scheduled an appointment with a specialist in esophageal issues at the Mayo Clinic, as a precaution.

My husband and I were sitting in the waiting room when Dr. Walters walked in with a huge bundle of papers in his hand, my medical records. He introduced himself and said he was almost sure my problem was low gastric acid, so he wanted me to have the Heidelberg test done before our appointment. The test involved swallowing a capsule that measures acid levels and transmits the information back to a computer. There was no string attached to the capsule, just a little metal transmitter pill. I swallowed it and within a few minutes the location signal appeared on the computer screen. The technician measured my pH level, which was normal, very low and acidic, as it should be. He then gave me half a cup of sodium bicarbonate (baking soda) to drink. The pH went up immediately. A normal stomach takes about 20 minutes to re-acidify, but we waited for almost an hour. My stomach simply wasn't making any acid. I felt overjoyed. I didn't have gastroparesis.

Dr. Walters said I could almost be diagnosed with achlorhydria, a condition in which the production of acid is completely absent. But he decided to wait longer than the test required and after one hour the pH finally started to go down. I had a severe case of hypochlorhydria, very low acid production.

———

Throughout the years, the little acid my stomach produced was enough to only partially digest food. That was the reason I had been experiencing digestive discomfort for a while. But when I was prescribed powerful acid blockers, my stomach could not even partially digest food anymore, and it simply started taking hours to get rid of content it should have digested in minutes. The main cause of my constant reflux was the amount of time food was left undigested in my stomach.

In spite of it all, I was extremely happy with the test results. Now I could do something about. The right treatment, for a change.

———

Low stomach acid is not an uncommon condition; diet, disease, and drugs, among other things, can cause it, and it gets worse with age. The older we get, the less acid our stomach produces. That is why it's mostly older people who suffer from acid reflux. In fact, the majority of cases of reflux, either heartburn or LPR, are caused by deficiency of acid, not excess. Unfortunately, most conventional doctors simply ignore decades of scientific research that show that low stomach acid is linked to a wide range of serious, chronic, and incurable diseases, including autoimmune diseases.

In recent years, the theory that leaky gut syndrome plays a part in autoimmunity has been gaining popularity in the scientific community. A recent study published by researchers at Lund University in Sweden has shown a connection between increased permeability of the intestines and multiple sclerosis. The study, done in mice infected with a disease similar to MS, showed that not only was the inflammatory response of leaky gut seen in the mice, but it also appeared to increase as multiple sclerosis progressed, with both conditions contributing to rising inflammation. Low stomach acid is considered a primary factor in leaky gut syndrome.[15]

One way that low stomach acid can contribute to an unhealthy gut is undigested food. Proteins and complex starches are digested and assimilated only with healthy levels of acid in the stomach. When these pass undigested out of the stomach, they become a feeding ground for harmful organisms like candida. As the balance of intestinal flora changes, digestion is affected and the lining of the gut weakens.

In addition, low stomach acid allows harmful bacteria to pass from the stomach into the intestines. When the stomach has enough acid, the acidic environment kills these bacteria swiftly. When the acid levels are too low, they survive and pass into the intestines where they cause many problems, including leaky gut syndrome.

Thankfully, low stomach acid is very easy to treat. I started by taking proteolytic enzymes with each meal, and soon after that I started supplementing with the acid itself – Betaine HCL. Dr. Walters instructed me to eat only solid foods and avoid drinking liquids with my meals. According to him, the liquid food suggested by the other doctor was diluting what little acid my stomach could make, and further compromising my digestion. It's no wonder I got so sick. The gastroenterologists had prescribed the exact opposite treatment of what I needed. Instead of acid supplements, powerful acid blockers. Instead of solid foods with no liquids around meal times, their recommendation was that I have only liquid foods.

After leaving Dr. Walters' clinic, I canceled the appointment at the Mayo Clinic and went back to Albuquerque. From the first day on the enzymes, I was able to start eating small portions of solid food without feeling bloated. Slowly the reflux got better. Symptoms such as the feeling of having a lump in my throat and the bitter taste on my mouth disappeared, my tongue turned from white to pink, and I started regaining my weight. The reflux resolved completely after I started taking the HCL supplement.

In most acid reflux cases, acid blockers cover up the symptoms. In my case, they didn't even cover up the symptoms because there was very little acid in my reflux. I was having mostly reflux of bile and other stomach contents. In the end, despite the difficult ordeal I went through, it was a good thing that the acid blockers didn't mask my symptoms. This way, I was forced to look for a solution and address the cause of the problem, instead of taking antacids every time I had a digestive discomfort.

After taking enzymes and HCL for three years, I noticed I could reduce the number of capsules with each meal without having any symptoms. I believe this means my stomach is producing more acid by itself. Dr. Walters had told me that this might happen, but there was no way of predicting if it would. So far, I have been able to reduce the amount of HCL and enzymes to half of what I was taking before. Since I started doing this simple treatment, I have never had an episode of acid reflux again. No matter what or how much I eat, my stomach can handle it. I tell my friends I now have the digestion I had when I was a teenager, and it's true.

Right before I had this problem, I was considering the idea of reintroducing meat in my diet. With this experience, I became aware of the importance of the digestive system to my health in general and specifically to the control of my multiple sclerosis. I learned that vegetarian diets are seen by many doctors as one of the main causes of low stomach acid, and I decided to take an extra step on my quest for a truly balanced diet, one that would be nutritious for my cells and good for my gut. I started centering my eating habits on whole foods. Presently I eat fish, seafood, chicken, red and organ meats, as well as eggs, lots of vegetables and some fruit. I try to eat organic and grass fed whenever possible. I reduced the amount of grains and gluten, and avoid sugar and processed foods. I also avoid dairy, since it's a requirement of the Coimbra Protocol. I believe that the changes I made in my diet might also be helping my stomach to produce acid again.

Through this whole ordeal, my multiple sclerosis remained in remission. I felt a little more tingling in my hands for a few months, but nothing that the MRIs detected, then or later. I was greatly relieved when I was able to start taking vitamin D again.

From the day I saw the first gastroenterologist to the day I saw Dr. Walters, less than two months had gone by, but to me if felt like a very long time. I still feel shocked beyond words when I think of what happened to me during those few weeks. All I needed was a couple of inexpensive supplements that can be found in any health store. Instead, I spent a small fortune in medical tests, lost a lot of weight in a short amount of time, had anxiety attacks thinking of the possibility of a gastroparesis diagnosis, was forced to stop taking vitamin D and therefore exposed to the risk of having a MS relapse, and missed many days of work. The most troublesome thing of all is to think that the gastroenterologists did nothing wrong in the eyes of conventional medicine. They followed the standard protocol. If you have acid reflux, you'll get a prescription for antacids.

I highly recommend that you instruct yourself further about this matter. As Dr. Wright says in his book, "low stomach acid is so common in any autoimmune condition that we are surprised when we don't find it. Correcting low stomach acid or other digestive malfunction can result in major improvement in the autoimmune disease."[16] Fixing this problem has taken my health to a whole new level, and that's why I decided to write this chapter and share this experience with you.

Chapter 7

"Because there are no profits to be made from selling natural treatments, the pharmaceutical industry, which controls the vast majority of medical research in the United States, will never investigate them or manufacture them. In fact, they will do everything possible to disparage them, because, should the word get out that they exist, natural treatments could threaten their stronghold on the practice of medicine."

– Dr. Jonathan V. Wright

A Word about Conventional Medications for MS

Let me start by saying that I'm not against conventional drugs for multiple sclerosis or for any other condition. On the contrary, I took copaxone for almost two years when I believed it might help me. After my MS diagnosis I took an antidepressant, which did wonders for my anxiety. When I had hope that even the acid blockers that caused me so much harm would alleviate my symptoms, I took them.

But when it comes to autoimmune diseases, I now know there is so much more we can do, using safer means to address the underlying causes of the problem, like chronic inflammation and resistance to vitamin D. My lack of trust of prescription medications for MS started with my own experience with copaxone, and deepened as I learned more about the drugs available today. Unfortunately, these drugs are not effective in delaying disability. They cut relapse rate, but there's no evidence that they can affect the long-term progression of the disease. In addition, they come with side effects that can be catastrophic, not to mention the ripple effect they create, causing secondary conditions that demand more medications, suppressing the immune system, and making it more difficult for the patient to recover, physically and mentally.

Recently, three independent studies looked at the effectiveness of the commonly used CRAB drugs (copaxone, rebif, avonex, betaseron). Notably, all three studies concluded that the CRABs have no significant effect on the long-term progression of disability.[17]

One of the studies[18] compared the disability progression of over 3,000 British patients who started receiving CRAB drugs in 2002 to the natural progression of untreated patients. The study found that not only there was no delay in disease progression for all the treatments; in fact, the disease progression was worse for patients who took the medications than for patients who received no treatment.

When it comes to the new generation of disease-modifying drugs for multiple sclerosis, immunosuppressants like gilenya, aubagio, or tysabri are apparently more effective than their predecessors at lowering the rate of relapses, but comparatively, they bring the risk of much more severe side effects, such as leukemia and PML (progressive multifocal leukoencephalopathy), among many others. Again, we don't know how effective these medications are in slowing down disease progression and accumulation of disability, or what other side effects they might bring with long term use.

One study that I find interesting is the clinical trial on the drug called anti-LINGO-1, a medication that might have the potential to reverse nerve demyelination. Phase II of the study has showed promising results with no significant side effects.[19] I believe it's a good thing that researchers are finally focusing on repairing the actual damage caused by multiple sclerosis. If we think about it, what makes life difficult for us are the symptoms caused from our damaged myelin, which no conventional drug has ever attempted to reverse.

However, when it comes to myelin repair, once again vitamin D seems to be ahead. As I write this, a new study on vitamin D and myelin regeneration has just been published.[20] In this study, researchers from the MS Society Cambridge Centre for Myelin Repair, identified that the vitamin D receptor protein pairs with an existing protein, called the RXR gamma receptor, already known to be involved in the repair of myelin. By adding vitamin D to brain stem cells where the proteins were present, they found the production rate of oligodendrocytes (myelin making cells) increased by 80 percent.

In one of his interviews, Dr. Coimbra makes a brief comparison between the effectiveness of conventional drugs and vitamin D in patients with autoimmune disorders. According to him, "Replenishing vitamin D in the doses required to achieve its beneficial effects implies restoring a natural mechanism, which allows patients to resume a normal life. It's a mechanism that nature took millions of years to develop, and even if the pharmaceutical industry spent centuries working on this issue, they would not get close to the benefits that vitamin D can provide to these patients."[21]

I do hope that in the near future scientists are able to develop a prescription medication that stops MS progression, with minimal side effects, even if only for the sake of patients who do not have access to unconventional treatments. But, at least for now, none of these drugs is an option that I'd consider for myself. Their risks are too great, and their benefits too questionable.

Chapter 8

"The desire and intention of someone who chooses to be a survivor and participate in their healing can provide results which far surpass what is expected."

– Dr. Bernie Siegel

Diet, Exercise, Stress Management

Diet

Vitamin D, when taken in the right amount, is capable of stopping the progression of aggressive autoimmune diseases. Still, if we are eating an excess of refined sugars, carbohydrates and trans fats, and our cells are not receiving the basic nutrition they require, can vitamin D keep us healthy indefinitely?

In truth, vitamin D in high doses is so effective that the great majority of patients on the Coimbra Protocol do not follow any specific diet, besides avoiding dairy. A few doctors who prescribe high doses of vitamin D recommend that patients avoid gluten. However, most doctors do not make this recommendation, including Dr. Coimbra.

After I quit the Best Bet Diet, I haven't felt the need of following any strict diet, but I do keep in mind that a lack of proper nutrients causes malfunctioning cells, and we need our cells as effective as they can be in combating our disease and its symptoms. Therefore, I now choose to eat whole, organic foods that will nourish my cells. Vitamin D does its part, and I do mine. But I don't worry excessively if sometimes I eat things that are not exactly considered healthy.

As I mentioned earlier, for more than a decade of my life I was a vegetarian. This was before I found out I had MS. My main source of protein was soy, dairy, and beans. I thought I had a healthy diet, but looking back I see that my diet was based on grains, gluten and dairy, which are all highly inflammatory food sources. I believe that all those years as a vegetarian actually inflamed my system, and might even have been responsible for my hypochlorhydria. An inflammatory diet, coupled with a possible genetic predisposition for autoimmunity, my poor digestion due to low stomach acid, and low levels of vitamin D, probably ensured that my predisposition turned into a full-blown disease.

I'm no longer a vegetarian, and based on what I've learned since my diagnosis, I would not be a vegetarian again. Presently, I've introduced many paleo principles in my diet. The Wahls Protocol, by Dr. Terry Wahls, is another book I recommend to everyone with an autoimmune disorder. Even if you don't intend to rigorously follow the diet recommended there, it gives wonderful insight in what a nutritious diet looks like. As a parenthesis, let me say that hypothetically, if one day I felt vitamin D was not enough to keep my MS in remission, I'd commit to a diet like the Wahls Protocol fully, as an extra support for my treatment. I do believe it's possible to achieve great results with the correct diet. For now, the Coimbra Protocol has kept my immune system very well balanced, even with much more flexible eating habits than what is usually required by diets for autoimmune conditions.

One thing that is important to mention is that I don't experience any symptoms when I eat grains, sugar or gluten, or any kind of processed foods. I avoid those foods, but I don't experience digestive discomforts or MS symptoms when I have them.

I can tolerate almost any food so well because I corrected my deficiency of stomach acid, which is a direct cause of food allergies and intolerances. Also, my vitamin D levels are adequate and, consequently, thousands of functions in my body are now working properly. And I do eat nutritious foods most of the time.

When it comes to this topic, I believe that making sure our gut is working properly is as important as improving our diet. Otherwise, we can eat foods dense in nutrients and still have serious deficiencies if our body can't digest them well.

Exercise

If you are following the Coimbra Protocol and you are able to exercise, you need to do at least 30 minutes of cardio exercises a day, five days a week, to avoid losing bone mass. According to Dr. Coimbra, patients that are mobile should start a cardio program right after their second appointment, when fatigue is usually gone.

In my particular case, I've noticed a few things since I started doing 30 – 45 minutes of cardio, five days a week. I'm now at my ideal weight without any need to watch my calories, I feel more energized in the days I work out, my mood is improved, and I feel it's much easier to keep anxiety under control.

Besides helping with our overall health, cardio exercises are also a great way to keep inflammation levels down. When we have an autoimmune disease it's important to start with whatever form of exercise is possible, even if only for a few minutes a day. There are great resources online, books and DVDs with work out programs developed specifically for patients with multiple sclerosis, rheumatoid arthritis, lupus, and so on. The main thing is to get up and move as well as we can. Every little bit is good for our body.

Stress Management

According to Dr. Coimbra, chronic stress, anxiety and depression are some of the main factors that may weaken the results of high-dose vitamin D. Autoimmune diseases and emotional stress are closely related, since one exacerbates the other's symptoms. Having an autoimmune condition in itself is a trigger to anxiety and stress, and persistent stress triggers autoimmunity, creating a vicious cycle. A high amount of stress hormones circulating in our blood stream for long periods can activate our immune system, damage our neurons, and lead to excess inflammation in the body and in the brain. It's known that about 80 percent of all multiple sclerosis relapses happen after episodes of intense stress.

Previously I mentioned a few tools I have used to deal with anxiety and stress, such as counseling, acupuncture, and an anti-depressant medication. Through counseling, I not only overcame my severe anxiety but also broke negative thought patterns and gained much needed self-knowledge, which helped me to become a more centered, more confident and positive person. Our mental states have great effect on the physical body, and I believe that when I understood how truly connected my mind and body are, it became easier to take the necessary steps toward improving my overall health.

One additional thing that I found to be of great help is having a project, a cause dear to our heart, or even a hobby. Something that we enjoy spending time on, and that can take our attention away from problems, even if only for a short while. A few months into my diagnosis, I restarted writing a novel I had been working on when I first got sick. Looking back, I realize that dedicating myself to that task kept my thoughts away from the disease for much of the time, and made it easier to keep my anxiety at bay. I strongly believe that finding something that gives us joy and spending time doing it can tremendously improve our physical and emotional health.

Along the years, I have also tried meditation, yoga, hypnosis. All these things combined helped me in different phases of my life, but I feel that what really pushed me towards where I'm today was the fact that I became completely engaged in my own healing process. Always looking for solutions, and not giving up. There are many different ways of learning how to cope with emotional imbalances. Choose whichever you think works best for you, but don't ignore it. Learning how to identify the signs of stress and anxiety, and not allowing them to take over your life, is an important step to maintaining your autoimmune disease in remission.

Chapter 9

"When we're courageous enough to be with what scares us,
we can awaken our intuition and create a new path for healing."

– Kris Carr

Your Own Journey

It might take years, maybe decades, until the medical community determines that high doses of vitamin D is the safest, most effective way to stop the progression of autoimmune diseases and even reverse the damage that has already been done. In my own personal journey, I learned very early that I didn't have years, much less decades, to wait for the perfect solution – a highly effective treatment that was proven and vetted by the scientific community. I had to find what was already out there, the best possible solution.

What I found has changed my life, and I know that millions of people around the world can benefit from this information as well. If you think high-dose vitamin D is something you'd like to try, at the end of the book, in Resources you'll find a list of discussion groups, videos, blogs and sites where you can interact with other patients, solve doubts about this treatment, find the updated list of doctors, and watch subtitled interviews with Dr. Coimbra.

Maybe you think it'll be difficult to find a doctor who follows the Coimbra Protocol in your country, but bear in mind that most doctors that are now prescribing high doses of vitamin D in Europe, Canada, and the US, were first introduced to this treatment by their own patients. Maybe your doctor will become interested, as well.

I really encourage you to join the discussion groups I listed in Resources. There are many knowledgeable members in those groups, including doctors who have autoimmune diseases and have chosen the Coimbra Protocol as their treatment. There, you'll be able to solve most doubts you might have about taking high doses of vitamin D. Don't be daunted by the language barrier. The groups have automatic translation for all posts and comments, and they have grown so big, with patients from so many parts of the world, that you can ask a question in any language and be sure to get an answer. Just a few years ago, having this level of interaction with patients from the other side of the ocean was not possible. My advice to you is that you use this to your advantage. Look for stories of people who overcame the same illness you have, introduce yourself, and talk to them. Use your critical sense to discover what might work for you. Take charge of your health.

Once you make the decision and start following the protocol, be persistent. I've seen people that started feeling better in a few weeks, and others, like me, that required a few months. Don't expect a miracle, for this is a medical treatment. Remember that most autoimmune diseases were many years in the making before the first symptoms manifested. Your body needs time to reverse decades of malfunctioning cells. For patients with multiple sclerosis, it's important to know that the central nervous system is the slowest system in the body to heal, so patience and determination are a must. When I talk to patients that are just starting the treatment, I tell them to make sure they are doing everything correctly, following through with lab tests and necessary adjustments of doses, and trying to keep a positive attitude during this process. After one year, when they get their MRIs (or the tests pertinent to their condition), they'll have solid evidence of what vitamin D can do.

So far, this has been my journey with an autoimmune disease. High doses of vitamin D brought relief from my symptoms, helped me get off a toxic medication, and allowed me to live without fear for what the future might bring. I have multiple sclerosis, but now I have my life back as well. I feel energized, I feel healthy, and I feel good most of the time. Feeling good is my normal. I know this is just the beginning. It can be your beginning too.

Chapter 10

"One of the most effective ways to neutralize medical pessimism is to find someone who had the same problem you do and is now healed."

– Dr. Andrew Weil

Testimonies

Larissa M.
Ouro Fino, Brazil
Multiple Sclerosis

I had the diagnosis of multiple sclerosis in 1999, when I was 30 years old, and began treatment with interferon beta right away. I was on the interferon for one year and during that period I had many flare ups. I also suffered with the medication's side effects. I soon realized that that drug was making me worse. My MRIs showed so many lesions that the doctors told me I'd likely be in a wheelchair in five years. I am a lawyer and at the time I worked for a law firm in a small town, so I decided to move to the city of São Paulo to see if I could find a better treatment.

I started following a macrobiotic diet and doing acupuncture sessions, as well as a few other alternative therapies. I decided not to take any prescription medication and just follow the alternative treatments. Unfortunately, those treatments didn't give me good results, and in 2004 I started taking copaxone, but I didn't feel improvements with copaxone either. This went on until 2005, when I heard about the treatment with high doses of vitamin D from a friend whose mother was a patient of Dr. Cicero Coimbra. I decided to schedule an appointment.

In my first appointment, Dr. Cicero gave me an amazing lecture on the role of vitamin D in the immune system, and I remember I finally relaxed on my chair, sitting there listening to him. I had been searching for years for something that made sense in this disease, and that day I knew I had found it. I thought to myself, "I am saved! This is the way."

When I told my family that I would start the treatment with vitamin D, they were concerned because at the time there were no support groups or a whole lot of literature for them to understand what the treatment was all about. They had to rely on my words alone, that I truly believed that the treatment was safe and effective.

I started the Coimbra Protocol in 2005 and fatigue was the first symptom to disappear. However, my level of resistance to vitamin D was very high and for the first two years I had problems absorbing it. Dr. Cicero said that my high levels of stress made this problem even worse. He suggested I take an anxiolytic for anxiety and stress, but I decided to search for spiritual help instead. I went to a very well-known spiritual healer in Brazil, John of God, in a place called "Casa de Dom Inácio de Loyola." I was surprised by the beauty of the work they did, and decided to live there for a while. After a few months, Dr. Cicero told me that finally, for the first time, my body was reacting and my resistance to vitamin D was overcome. The improvements started to come, slowly.

After I had lived at "Casa de Dom Inácio de Loyola" for a year and a half, John of God told me I was cured of MS, and right after that, Dr. Cicero told me that my vitamin D levels were fine and that I wouldn't have flare ups or disease progression anymore. The improvements kept coming, and after 10 years I feel I'm still improving. About two years ago I noticed that my intolerance to heat was gone. I live in a very hot state in Brazil, but now I can get out and walk in the streets even on hot days. I also had bladder incontinence, and just recently I noticed that the leakages are not happening anymore. I no longer have to wear protective underwear! I still have a few problems, such as urinary urgency and difficulty bending my left leg. I think that if I didn't have those problems I would not remember that I had MS. I feel I'm cured. I've been on high doses of vitamin D for over 10 years. I've never had a side effect from this treatment, and I've never had a relapse again.

One interesting thing is that right after I started my treatment, my mother also had an appointment with Dr. Cicero and started taking high doses of vitamin D to treat a health problem. My mom was 80 years old when she started her treatment. Now she is 91 years old, she takes 60,000 IU daily and does regular tests to make sure her calcium levels and kidney functions are fine. Recently she received the news from her geriatrician that her kidneys are in excellent shape. Another advantage I found in this treatment is that my immune system is so much stronger now. I don't get colds or urinary infections as I used to, and this also helps with keeping MS in remission.

I have a video made by my physical therapist some years ago, when I walked with difficulty. Soon I will make a new video and post it in our support group, showing the improvements I've made in the last years. It's been 17 years since I was diagnosed with MS. In the past 10 years my disease has stopped progressing, and instead of getting worse, I'm recovering.

Nayra B.
(Written by her mother, Marcia C.)
São Paulo, Brazil
Multiple Sclerosis

My daughter, Nayra, has multiple sclerosis.

Today this fact no longer scares me, but 16 years ago MS was my worst nightmare, because when she was 10 years old, Nayra had her first flare up. It started in April of 2000, with tingling in the fingers of her right hand. I took her to the pediatrician and he told us it was nothing, we shouldn't worry. Three days later the tingling had increased and I then took her to the emergency room. They requested many tests, blood tests, urine, ultrasound, MRIs, and finally the tests showed a lesion in the cervical, between C3 and C4. The doctors suspected a tumor and suggested surgery might be necessary, but I decided to get a second opinion and took her to a different hospital. Those were very difficult days for us. She started treatment with corticosteroids and anti-inflammatory for 6 months. She improved rapidly and soon she had recovered completely.

Almost a year went by and in 2001 the tingling started again, this time in the lower extremities, beginning in the feet and climbing up to the legs quickly. I was shocked and rushed her to the ER. We went through the same thing all over again, several tests and more corticosteroids. This time the doctors spoke of "demyelinating disease", but we still didn't get a diagnosis.

And then came 2002, when she had two relapses, and 2003, when she had two relapses more. And each relapse brought a different symptom. Tingling in the arms, legs and abdomen, feeling heat or cold in different parts of the body, and finally vision problems. In one of the relapses in 2003, Nayra partially lost her vision. I panicked. I took her to the hospital, carrying with me all her medical records. The neurologist who saw her told me she had multiple sclerosis. I didn't know what multiple sclerosis was. I was so terrified that the more the doctor explained, the less I understood. She was hospitalized to take steroids. With this diagnosis, I went to "Hospital das Clínicas", in São Paulo, where I knew she would be treated by MS specialists. The neurologist prescribed copaxone, a painful injection she had to take every day. This was very difficult for a 13 year old.

I started researching the disease, and the more information I found the more frightened I became. I went to MS associations but I always left those places very depressed, because I saw many people in wheelchairs and with various disabilities. I imagined my daughter in that situation in a few years, and despaired. I was having a hard time going on with my life, my work, and dealing with the idea that my daughter had a serious, incurable illness. I asked God daily for a blessing and a light in those dark times. One day, in Hospital das Clínicas, I met a neurologist who also had multiple sclerosis. She was an assistant to Nayra's neurologist. At that time, this doctor already had severe disabilities. She couldn't walk without the aid of canes, and spoke with difficulty. That day she told me that that was the future of patients with MS. But she also gave me the name of a Yahoo group, where I could get answers to my many questions. This was a group of MS patients who were treated at that hospital. I joined the group that same day, introduced myself and talked about Nayra's problems with MS. I left my phone number, asked for help, a word, any comfort to my heart.

A few days later there was a message on my voice mail from a woman who also had a daughter with MS, and her story was similar to mine. Her daughter had been diagnosed at a very early age as well, and the whole family had suffered a lot. She asked me to call her so we could talk about this neurologist, Dr. Cicero Coimbra, who had started a new treatment for MS, with vitamin D. I called her, and she told me that when she found out her daughter had MS, she had contacted 50 of the most reputable neurologists in Brazil, all well-known professors and head of departments in the main hospitals in the country. Only one of those doctors answered her, Dr. Cicero Coimbra. I marveled at what she told me, about the treatment with vitamin D and the results her daughter was having. I called Dr. Cicero's office and scheduled an appointment right away. Our first visit lasted almost four hours, with detailed explanations of the treatment and what we could expect from it. We left full of hope, and with a prescription for vitamin D and some other supplements. As soon as we left the appointment, Nayra said she would never take the injections again. Dr. Cicero had told us that it made no difference if she kept taking copaxone or not; it was up to us. Vitamin D would balance Nayra's immune system, and the disease would go into remission.

This was in 2003. Nayra has been on high doses of vitamin D for 13 years now. Dr. Cicero was right. She has never taken another injection or steroids, and the best part is that she has never had a relapse again. Over the months, I realized that Nayra's fatigue was gone; she enrolled in the school's indoor soccer team. She started walking to school again, I didn't need to drive her anymore. Our lives began to change in every way. I began to sleep better, work better, and feel better as well. In short, everything improved. When I told Dr. Cicero that Nayra was taking part in her soccer team's championships, even he was surprised at how quickly she was recovering.

At first we had appointments with Dr. Cicero every three months, then every six months, and finally annual visits. Thus the years passed, with dose adjustments, regular lab tests, taking the supplements, following the specific diet required by the protocol, and most importantly, taking vitamin D.

Normal life!

During these years, Dr. Cicero did not request MRIs, for Nayra was always well. When she was 18 she lived for two years in Italy by herself, and never had any symptoms. She goes through her life as any other young woman; she studies, works, travels, rides her bike, does sports, goes to the gym. And take her vitamins. One recommendation that Dr. Cicero really insisted upon was that she should do everything possible to avoid stress, because stress and anxiety can trigger relapses. With vitamin D and no stress, there's been no relapses for all these 13 years. Nayra has a completely normal life. She's a beautiful, lively, healthy young woman.

In the beginning of 2015, Dr. Cicero requested MRIs so we could compare them to the previous images. And what a good surprise it was, for all the lesions on her brain and spinal cord were gone! There was only a small, almost imperceptible lesion on the brain. It's so sad that most doctors seem determined to remain in ignorance when it comes to this treatment. Whenever possible, I talk about Nayra's experience with vitamin D to people with MS and to everyone who has an autoimmune disease.

Thousands of people are following this treatment and improving every day.

People around the world are coming to Brazil or consulting with doctors in other countries that are already prescribing this protocol. As always, I'm grateful to God for giving me this grace and putting me in contact with Dr. Cicero Galli Coimbra. I'm eternally grateful to Dr. Cicero for his dedication and faithfulness to the Hippocratic Oath, for his dedication to his studies and his patients, the contribution he made to medicine and science, and the human being he is, giving part of his life to give us health. Thank you Dr. Cicero Galli Coimbra.

Leila G.
Divino, Brazil
Psoriasis and Psoriatic Arthritis

I felt the first symptoms of psoriasis about 20 years ago. It started in my scalp, with itching and flaking of the skin, which I thought was dandruff. I went to a general practitioner who prescribed an ointment, which I used for a while but it just made it worse. After that I went to a number of doctors; however, I didn't get a diagnosis. I had no idea what was wrong with me.

In 1992 I got married, and by then some small lesions had appeared in my back as well. Around that time I experienced a serious emotional trauma, and I believe that was what triggered the first major flare up of the disease. Psoriasis took over my body. Even my nails developed lesions and started to fall. Sometimes the lesions hurt, the skin cracked and bled, especially when I was nervous. Only my feet and hands were free of lesions. Wherever I went, I left flakes of skin on the ground. My family, especially my mother, was not supportive. I think she wanted a perfect daughter.

Thankfully, my husband was very understanding and supportive, and in the midst of all my health issues, we had three daughters. Meanwhile, I finally got a diagnosis of psoriasis. I'm a grade school teacher and my job was very demanding. Add to that many family crises (my mother even said once that I had the devil in my body, because of the psoriasis) and the problems of everyday life, which made the disease worse.

In 2003 my dermatologist prescribed the drug methotrexate. At first everything was fine and my skin cleared in less than a month. But when I stopped the medication I got psoriatic arthritis as a rebound effect. Oh yes. Now I was very sick, in severe pain, with small daughters and almost unable to walk. My family was no help, quite the opposite; my mother used to open her bible and say that Jesus was talking to her and that I was suffering like that because I had too many sins. Such was the support I had. My husband took care of our daughters and me by himself, besides doing all the heavy work in our land.

The treatment was difficult. I live in a very small town in Brazil where there were no rheumatologists. I had to go to a bigger town to get my treatment with prednisone and diclofenac. At the time, I did not know all the side effects those drugs could cause. I got very swollen, my skin got even worse than it was before, and that was the worst time of my life. I put myself in God's hands and asked Him for a cure, because I knew those treatments would never be a cure. I spent two years unable to work and had to take leave from my students because of the arthritis.

One day, when I was in another city waiting for a doctor's appointment for one of my daughters, I became very sick. I vomited all night and had to be taken to the emergency room. It was my body rejecting all the medications. I decided it was time to stop taking those drugs and began to search for alternative treatments. I was still taking indomethacin, though, which had been prescribed by another rheumatologist. Later I stopped that as well.

I began to treat myself with homeopathy, herbs, and exercises. Slowly I started to feel better and was able to go for short walks. While taking prednisone I had gone from 155 to 200 pounds, so I started dieting and lost the extra weight. I eventually started practicing Capoeira in 2010, Pilates in 2013, and in May 2014 I started practicing Muay Thay. I do not know what exactly brought the improvements for the arthritis, it was probably a combination of everything I did – quitting the prescription drugs, taking homeopathy and natural treatments, losing weight, and exercising. I felt I was pulling myself together, but my skin was still very bad and filled with lesions. In the middle of my quest, I found a group on Facebook called "Psoriase." Some of the members talked about their experience with natural treatments, and one of them started sharing with us her experience with a "treatment with high doses of vitamin D." In this journey, God has always found a way of putting angels in my life.

I got interested and started researching. The members that knew this treatment were adamant about how good it was. In August 2014, I started taking 10,000 IU of vitamin D a day and continued my research. I decided to call Dr. André Lage, in the town of Vespasiano. Then, he was the only doctor in the state of Minas Gerais that prescribed the protocol created by Dr. Cicero Coimbra. At that time I could not afford to see him, but I decided to save my money and invest in my health. I had to get rid of that disease. In December of 2014 I finally had my appointment.

Because the doctor was in a different city, the day of my appointment I left my home at 1:30 am and got back at 8 pm. I had the best doctor's consultation of my life. It lasted two and a half hours. We talked about many different topics, Dr. André asked me all about the psoriasis, and explained the treatment in detail. I had already done the necessary lab tests, since Dr. André had sent me the request for the tests by email, prior to the appointment. I left his office feeling certain that this would be the treatment of my life. He prescribed 70,000 IU of vitamin D, glutamine to help heal my cartilages, and a compound with a number of other vitamins and supplements.

Amazingly, the improvements started immediately. My skin began to clear. Only my family knew I was on this treatment. I had not told anyone about it, but people's reaction was not long in coming. My appointment happened during the summer vacation, but when I returned to work in February, my colleagues began to compliment me and ask what I was doing. People were noticing how much better I looked. And best of all, I no longer left skin flakes wherever I went.

Today, one year after my first appointment and a year and four months since the day I started taking vitamin D, the improvement is astounding. My skin keeps getting better. This is the treatment I asked God for. And I will not keep this a secret. I want to do for others what was done for me.

I'm so grateful to all the angels that helped me along the way. Dr. Cicero Coimbra, Dr. André Lage, the members of the Facebook group who encouraged me to learn more about high doses of vitamin D, the holistic therapists with whom I've worked along the years, and so many others.

Thank you.

Ana L.
Bucharest, Romania
Multiple Sclerosis

I had the first symptoms of MS in 2008, but I was diagnosed only one year later. I remember that one day I was at the airport and at some point I just couldn't walk anymore. My small pink suitcase was suddenly so heavy; I cancelled my flight and returned home. As I got some rest, the symptoms went away.

The next day I went to the hospital and as soon as I started to recount my experience, the doctor asked for tests. The MRI and the lumbar puncture confirmed the MS diagnosis. Of course, I suffered a lot; it was a shock. It was so difficult to accept such a terrible diagnosis, especially at such a young age as mine. I was in my early twenties.

I began the treatment with interferon beta, but a few months later that same year I had new lesions, confirmed by the MRI. I had a poor response to this medication, as I continued to have a number of relapses every year. I usually had two or three relapses in a year. The treatment with methylprednisolone helped me every time to reach almost a complete recovery of my symptoms, but never quite a full recovery.

Then, at the beginning of 2012 I had the strongest, most aggressive relapse ever. I took eight grams of solumedrol, one gram per day during eight days. I had a modest recovery with the cortisone treatment and a few sessions of physical therapy. A new MRI confirmed the presence of four new lesions on the spinal cord. I was really sick for more than a year. Walking was a huge effort during that period; I had new symptoms like the "MS hug", equilibrium problems, and a serious spasticity.

So, in that short period of time I reached an EDSS (Expanded Disability Status Scale) of 4.5. My MS was considered very aggressive and I began a treatment with tysabri, a monoclonal antibody, a very efficient drug, but with serious side effects, including PML. I was positive to the JC virus, so my neurologist, an MS specialist, told me that I could not take it for more than two years. I took this drug for almost a year. It was my personal choice to stop it in 2013.

What I had not told my neurologist was that in 2012, after my relapse, I had begun taking vitamin D. In April of 2012 I started reading the studies published on Pubmed, a service of the US National Library of Medicine. So many studies confirmed the importance of vitamin D for this disease. I began taking physiological, safe doses, between 5,000 – 10,000 units daily. I remember that a study of Dr. Mowry impressed me. The study, published on Pubmed, said that each 10 ng/ml increase in the vitamin D levels was associated with a 15 percent lower risk of a new T2 lesion and a 32 percent lower risk of a relapse.

One day I read a book where I found some information that grabbed my attention, about a neurologist from Brazil who was treating MS with high doses of vitamin D. I watched a documentary of a young Brazilian patient, Daniel Cunha, named "Vitamina D – Por Uma Outra Terapia."

I did more research about this doctor and his treatment, and I came into contact via Internet with his MS patients. His name was Cicero Galli Coimbra MD, PhD, neurologist, head of the lab of Neuropathology and Neuroprotection and also professor of Neurology at the Federal University of São Paulo.

And so begins the good part of the story.

Briefly, at this moment I have been following Dr. Coimbra's protocol for three years and seven months. I am currently taking 70,000 units of vitamin D daily, associated with a low calcium diet and an abundant hydration to avoid hypercalcemia and hypercalciuria. My dose was adjusted last year, in my last appointment with Dr. Coimbra in Brazil.

This dose of vitamin D was determined based on my individual lab tests' results. I have not had any side effects with this treatment. I have blood and urine tests done every four months and they confirm that my kidneys are healthy.

I now have an EDSS of 3, and I've had significant improvements in my motor symptoms and my equilibrium. The urinary urgency improved by 90 percent. The spasticity and the "MS hug" disappeared completely, and the quality of my life is greatly improved.

Around three years ago, Dr. Coimbra told me that I'd not experience any other relapse, that I'd have a normal life, except for the disabilities acquired when I had active MS, from which I may progressively recover with physical therapy. I believe that he was right, because my MS has not been active anymore, the last MRIs done in 2013 and 2015 confirmed that the disease is stable, without new or active lesions. I think I am quite lucky because I had the opportunity to discover and start this treatment. My goal for this year is to achieve better control of my emotions and to deal better with stress. Sometimes, when I am very stressed, some old symptoms temporarily return.

As I live in Europe, going to Brazil for consultations is definitely a big effort, but it's worth it. This is a very low-cost and effective treatment. And there is a great difference in my life before and after high doses of vitamin D. The words cannot entirely describe the gratitude and respect I have for Dr. Coimbra and the work he's been doing for the last 13 years.

Juliana H.
Rio de Janeiro, Brazil
Rheumatoid Arthritis

It all started in April of 2014, when after feeling pain in my joints for a short while, I was diagnosed with rheumatoid arthritis. I was 38 years old at that point, and I had over 20 inflamed joints.

I was walking with great difficulty, I could not drive, I could not open a carton of milk or a bottle of water, it was very hard for me to get dressed, and I could not even do the dishes because it was impossible to lift pots and pans. But my greatest fear was not being able to take care of my son, who was five at the time. I could barely put his shoes on when he was getting ready for school.

Still, I was confident I would get better. I was being treated by one of the most reputable rheumatologists in Rio de Janeiro, and I was optimistic. I started the standard treatment prescribed by the doctor, but not long after I began to despair because I realized that I would have to take very strong medications for the rest of my life. Then I joined some RA online groups and noticed that the conventional treatment still left most patients feeling pain, not to mention the side effects. Luckily, I had heard about the high-dose vitamin D treatment. My sister-in-law had just been diagnosed with multiple sclerosis, and because of that, I had watched an interview with Dr. Cicero Coimbra about the subject. I did a lot of research, talked to many patients, and read many scientific articles. Therefore, when I decided to seek this treatment I was very well informed. The only thing that bothered me a bit was the lack of patients with rheumatoid arthritis following the Coimbra Protocol. At that time, there were very few, and this made me wonder if the treatment would be as effective for RA as it was for MS. Still, I scheduled an appointment with Dr. Sergio Menendez, a physician from Dr. Coimbra's staff, in São Paulo.

I had decided to follow both treatments simultaneously, vitamin D and the conventional therapy, but after two months of taking methotrexate and prednisone, I rethought my decision. Methotrexate made me very ill on the day of application and the next day; I pretty much did nothing those days. Prednisone helped, but I was too scared to take it for a long time, because I have an aunt who also suffers from an autoimmune condition and she took steroids for a long time, and after 10 years, she needed a hip replacement as a consequence of the steroids. But the final straw for me was when I started feeling pain in areas of my body that I had never felt before, mainly back pain. I found out that it was not the disease that was causing it, but the medication. One of methotrexate's side effects was back pain! Suddenly, conventional treatment started not making sense to me. A drug that should take my pain away was causing me more pain, besides weakening my immune system. I quit methotrexate. I kept taking the low-dose prednisone while I waited for my appointment with Dr. Menendez, which would be in a month.

I started my treatment with vitamin D in August. In the first month the fatigue, which I had not even realized was a symptom of the RA, improved a lot. Slowly I started working out again, and by my doctor's advice, I started taking ballet classes, which I love and had already done for 15 years when I was a child. At first I'd go limping to the class; I was in a lot of pain and could not even do half of the exercises, but gradually I got better, and by November I was able to follow the whole class. In December, I was doing and feeling great!

Seeing the effect that high doses of vitamin D had on me, allowing me to get rid of powerful painkillers and most importantly, taking my pain away, I became eternally grateful to Dr. Coimbra. Today, I feel obliged to talk about this treatment, so that it reaches more and more people, and brings relief to patients with rheumatoid arthritis who are still suffering from the disease and the drugs. I and some other patients that follow the Coimbra Protocol have created a group on Facebook to exchange experiences about the treatment in rheumatic autoimmune diseases, especially rheumatoid arthritis. I also began to post photos in yoga postures, for I started practicing yoga in the beginning of 2015, as a support for my treatment. Yoga has now become another way for me to show the results I'm having with this protocol, and to encourage those who are still unsure or just starting the treatment.

My latest blood tests, CRP and ESR, show no inflammation whatsoever. I hope that one day the Coimbra Protocol is recognized as an official treatment for autoimmune diseases, because it can ease the suffering for many patients. Only those who go through an experience with this disease know the pain we feel, both physically and mentally. I will always be available to share my experience and the results I'm having with high doses of vitamin D.

Fabiana G.
São Paulo, Brazil
Primary Progressive Multiple Sclerosis

In 1992 I started experiencing some strange symptoms. I had an episode of facial paralysis, and occasionally I experienced dizziness, vertigo, and numbness throughout different parts of my body. But since these symptoms always coincided with stressful situations, I assumed it was just stress and did not pay much attention to them. In 2008 things got worse and I started having problems walking due to a lack of balance, and sometimes my legs would "lock". I also felt fatigue, numbness, hypersensitivity in the sole of my feet, and blurred vision. I got pregnant and during the pregnancy, all these symptoms went away, but soon after having my baby they came back. Numbness, tingling, heaviness in my legs, blurred vision and sometimes bladder and bowel incontinence. As my stress level worsened, the intensity of the symptoms worsened as well. The connection between my emotional state and these symptoms has always been clear to me. Still, I didn't want to believe I had anything serious, so I just tried a variety of alternative therapies, but nothing seemed to help.

I finally went to a neurologist in 2011. He asked for a brain MRI, which showed three minor lesions. The report didn't mention anything about demyelinating disease. The doctor then requested a spinal cord MRI but I did not do it right away. The symptoms were gradually getting worse. I researched it on Google and it looked like multiple sclerosis.

I went to a different neurologist, and just with the clinical exam and the brain MRI, he diagnosed me with multiple sclerosis. He explained about the conventional treatment and its side effects, and told me I would have quality of life for about 15 years, but not to worry, because medicine was always advancing and nowadays there were some very functional wheelchairs...

Fast forward to neurologist number three. Based on the brain MRI and his examination, he didn't think I had MS. He asked for a number of tests, he suspected I had Devic's disease. I had spinal cord MRIs done, which showed extensive lesions in the cervical, thoracic and lumbar spine. I also had a number of active lesions. I finally realized how serious my situation was! The brain lesions were unchanged from the previous MRI, but the report now pointed to demyelinating disease. The results were indicative of Devic's disease or transverse myelitis. I then had a spinal tap done and it was positive for oligoclonal bands. I did a series of blood tests, including FAN and aquaporin 4, which were negative.

These results ruled out Devic's, but the neurologist decided to order all the tests again, for he still believed that's what I had. Around that same time, one of my sisters saw an interview with Dr. Coimbra where he talked about the treatment with high doses of vitamin D for autoimmune diseases. She got interested, researched about it, and called his office to schedule an appointment for me. I had my first appointment with Dr. Coimbra in June 12, 2012. My appointment lasted three hours, and it was an amazing consultation. Dr. Coimbra diagnosed me with primary progressive multiple sclerosis, and I started the treatment right away.

A few days later, neurologist number three contacted me. The results of my second round of tests had come back, and Devic's disease was completely ruled out. He said that we should start the treatment for MS. Well, it was too late. I had already started my treatment for MS.

It has been three years and seven months since I started taking high doses of vitamin D. I still feel some of the symptoms, due to the lesions I have on my spinal cord, but everything is much improved. The blurred vision is completely gone, my left leg feels heavy sometimes but doesn't "lock" anymore, I can tolerate heat better than I used to, the incontinence problem is almost gone, and I can walk much better as well.

As for my latest MRIs, the results are unbelievable. All my large cervical lesions have completely disappeared! The comparison of these images with the previous MRIs is simply amazing. Two of the brain lesions have also disappeared, there was only one left, almost imperceptible. The thoracic lesions are reduced in size, and since I started the treatment, I have had no new lesions.

Because I still few some symptoms, in my last appointment my vitamin D dose was adjusted to 180,000 IU per day. I hope to keep improving. This treatment is effective and so easy to follow, especially when we consider what it gives us. I've gotten so much better, and with no side effects.

Leila M.
Coqueiral, Brazil
Crohn's Disease and Ankylosing Spondylitis

In 2008, I was diagnosed with Crohn's disease. But to arrive at this diagnosis, I had to travel a long and arduous path. In my first visit to the proctologist, he thought I had a sexually transmitted disease. I told him my problem was not a sexually transmitted disease, since I had not had a blood transfusion, had never shared needles, and didn't have a lifestyle that could lead to a sexually transmitted disease. The doctor asked for a battery of tests, including HIV.

In this appointment, it was not possible to have a sigmoidoscopy exam, such was the inflammation in the area. The doctor prescribed antibiotics, analgesics, and an anti-inflammatory. I had no improvements and went to see him again the following week, but because the tests' results were not ready yet, he told me to keep taking the same drugs. At the time he thought I had some kind of infection, so he said he could not prescribe steroids because they would reduce my immunity, and according to him I needed all my antibodies to fight the infection.

About 20 days later, the tests' results came back. I didn't have a sexually transmitted disease. The proctologist then prescribed steroids, which minimized the inflammation. Nevertheless, there were many side effects, like insomnia, fluid retention, and acne. I continued using corticosteroids for about six months, and in this period I was finally diagnosed with Crohn's disease.

The corticosteroids eased my symptoms. There were times when the disease went into remission, and I felt well. But every year I had a crisis. And in 2012, the corticosteroids stopped being effective in controlling my crises. Crohn's had infiltrated my joints, causing arthritis; my kidneys, causing kidney stones; my esophagus, causing gastroesophageal reflux, and the large intestine, causing anal bleeding and continuous pain, as well as excessive gas and other conditions such as fissures, hemorrhoids and severe constipation.

I was very sick and my only option then was the treatment with adalimumab. But when I read all the side effects caused by this drug I refused to take it.

I prayed a lot, and asked God to show me another treatment. Once I got home from church I started searching on Google for an effective treatment with no side effects, something that could take the symptoms of Crohn's away. My prayers were answered, and God showed me the solution to the severe suffering I was in. I found an online group that talked about the treatment with high doses of vitamin D. I researched about it and decided to try, and with a month of use, all the symptoms mentioned above were gone.

But as autoimmune diseases can trigger other autoimmune diseases, just as I started taking vitamin D I was diagnosed with ankylosing spondylitis, a type of arthritis caused by Crohn's. I went to four rheumatologists. Three told me I could not do without the use of the medication and that I would stop walking if I did not start the conventional treatment as soon as possible. They gave me a period of 30 days to start treatment. In all my appointments, I mentioned I had started this treatment with vitamin D, and the importance of this vitamin in autoimmune diseases. All the doctors seemed interested.

It's been three years. I did not take the immunosuppressants, and I have never been so healthy as I am today. I now have quality of life, I can eat everything, nothing that I eat causes me harm, I do my housework, and I exercise again.

I feel very fortunate to have been graced with the knowledge of vitamin D. I no longer remember that I have Crohn's disease and ankylosing spondylitis.

I want to share my experience with everybody that also has these illnesses, and tell them to take courage and seek a painless treatment, without side effects. This treatment is vitamin D.

David N.
São Paulo, Brazil
Multiple Sclerosis

After many, many tests and visits to a number of doctors and neurologists, in late 2012 I was diagnosed with MS. For months I had felt dizziness and twisting of the mouth, my face used to tremble, and sometimes my reasoning and speech got confused. I thought the worst. I was 33 years old and very frightened at that time.

I started to read all I could about MS. My wife found an online group of people dealing with MS who followed a treatment with high doses of vitamin D, and they all seemed very satisfied with it. That was how I discovered the treatment with vitamin D. I was in the hospital taking steroids due to the relapse and the nurse was worried because I was glued to the computer all night long, reading everything I could about this treatment. I decided to start the Coimbra Protocol right away, less than one month after my diagnosis. I never did the conventional treatment. I read a lot about the conventional drugs as well, and chose to follow only the treatment with vitamin D.

I also changed my lifestyle a bit. I have a healthier diet now and try to avoid inflammatory foods, like sugar, fast food, sodas. I exercise and make sure I get plenty of sleep. In the first eight months of treatment I had some ups and downs. I knew it was common to have these fluctuations until vitamin D started to become effective and the disease stabilized. Ups and downs usually happen when we go through severe stress or are exposed to intense heat, so now I take precautions to avoid stress and heat. Since I started taking high doses of vitamin D I haven't had any flare ups, and I do not feel anymore that my body is unpredictable. I live without fear of relapses, I travel and work a lot, I skateboard, and today I can say that I feel better than I did before my diagnosis. I hope to continue this way.

What I say to those starting treatment with vitamin D is that it works, and it works very well. It might take a while, but as long as you have medical supervision, make the necessary dose adjustments and have patience, it will be effective. As a fellow patient says, "With high doses of vitamin D only the improvements are progressive."

At the time of my diagnosis I used to read the many positive stories in the group, how people recovered with the Coimbra Protocol, and always wondered if one day I would be able to say the same. Thank God I am! It's been over three years now, and I continue to do everything I did before my diagnosis. Actually, today I do more. I now have a one year old daughter at home and a job that's very demanding.

I had MRIs done in 2012, 2013 and 2014. In each test the results were better, with a slight decrease in the size of some lesions, and the complete disappearance of others. The fact is that in each MRI the number and size of my lesions gradually decreased. The next MRI is scheduled for the end of 2016. In my last visit with my doctor, in 2015, he said that the disease is totally stabilized. I just need to see him once a year from now on. All tests' results are fine, but since I'll continue taking high doses of vitamin D, I need to keep doing my regular checkups. Also, I need to keep the protocol diet with its basic restrictions. In short, I keep working hard, traveling, having fun, enjoying my baby daughter, and even dealing with the common problems of everyday life, without worrying about relapses and MS.

A curiosity: When I was diagnosed in 2012, I could not ride a bike due to the dizziness I felt. I thought I'd never be able to ride a motorcycle again, so I sold my bike that I loved. After about 8 months of treatment, I had improved so much that I bought another bike, and this time I got a motocross bike. I usually do motocross on Sundays, with jumps more than a meter high (okay, okay... amateur jumps), without MS getting in the way. The other riders have no idea I have MS.

I now have met several of the patients from whom I used to read the testimonies. I've met personally more than 50 people who follow the treatment with high doses of vitamin D and are very happy with it. In 2013 I also had the privilege of meeting Dr. Michael Holick, who was present at an event in São Paulo with Dr. Cicero Coimbra and many of his patients.

Good health to Dr. Cicero Coimbra and all the doctors that are prescribing this protocol! I hope that more and more people around the world have access to this treatment, and that more and more doctors become interested in this fantastic protocol. I also hope that everybody with MS has their vitamin D levels checked, since several studies report that lower levels of vitamin D are risk factors for the activity and progression of MS, and every day we see new studies linking vitamin D and the risk of MS relapses and disease progression. Although difficult, due to strong pressure from large pharmaceutical companies, I still have hopes that one day Vitamin D will be the first choice of treatment for autoimmune diseases, or at least that all patients who choose this treatment will have access to it. Good health to us all!

Dr. Cicero, thank you!

Yara C.
São Paulo, Brazil
Multiple Sclerosis

I have been a patient of Dr. Cicero Coimbra for nearly six years and follow his protocol to the letter. I got to him in appalling condition, with vision loss in the left eye (only saw 20 percent), speech and concentration problems, horrible tingling all over the body, trigeminal neuralgia, left arm and leg incoordination and the most serious symptom of all: a very strong vertigo that afflicted me 24 hours a day, seven days a week. I could barely go to the bathroom alone, and I used to fall even when using the walls for support. It was an indescribable feeling of falling in an elevator shaft, but backwards and with everything going around me in circles. I could not turn my head even when I was lying in bed. I was in this situation for several months.

At the time I was taking copaxone, which did not help, besides giving me terrible side effects. Since I was a pharmaceutical marketing professional for over 10 years, I knew exactly who was profiting from that drug, and it was not me. I was visibly getting worse.

I thought there had to be another alternative, and decided to go after it. It was then that I started searching and found a group of patients of Dr. Cicero Coimbra, at Yahoo Groups. I spent a couple of months reading their accounts of the treatment, asking questions and interacting with them. They showed me many scientific studies linking vitamin D to clinical improvement in patients with multiple sclerosis, and this definitely sparked my interest in this new therapy. I talked to some patients who were ready to answer all my questions, and then a new path began to emerge in my life.

I scheduled an appointment with Dr. Cicero; however, despite all the testimonies showing the therapeutic success of high doses of vitamin D and the broad scientific background that supported this new treatment, I was afraid. Taking a chance on the unknown is always difficult, and breaking our own paradigms is not an easy thing to do. After all, by leaving the conventional treatment I would be confronting the opinion of neurologists who, until then, I considered the best in my country. I knew that Dr. Cicero was not well-accepted among his fellow doctors because he had proposed a change; he had dared to step beyond the general consensus. But I also knew that those who dare to propose new ideas are usually ridiculed at first, even when there's clear evidence they tread a path of success and professional ethics.

I pondered a lot about all this before I finally went to the appointment. It was my life that was at stake and I did not intend to act on impulse and much less blindly. From the day of my first appointment on, a sunny future began to shine on my horizon, and a new story began. That doctor, with great and unexpected humility, although in a very forceful way, looked deep into my eyes and said, "Yara, the nightmare is over. You'll no longer have problems with multiple sclerosis."

I stopped taking copaxone during the first month of treatment.

A few months later, precisely seven months, I began to improve significantly. I started taking some steps on my own; one day I walked five meters, the next I walked 10 meters, then the next day it was already 20 meters. Sometimes even this small effort was too much and I had to spend a whole week at home, recovering. But I did not give up. I returned to work because I knew that my recovery also depended on my commitment and emotional balance. At that time, I had already seen a video of Dr. Cicero on YouTube, where he spoke about the impact of stress and anxiety in the aging process and in autoimmune diseases. He cited many important studies, widely consolidated in the scientific literature, and what he said made me ponder deeply about the patterns of behavior that I had systematically adopted along the years; patterns that simply put my immune system on alert and caused it to attack my own body. It was already clear to me that emotional control was a major factor on my recovery. I needed, more than ever, to control my anxiety.

In this interview that shed so much light on my internal conflicts, Dr. Cicero explained how ongoing stress blocks neurogenesis – the birth of new neurons. Therefore, if I wanted to be successful in the treatment I had chosen, I knew I should act on that precious scientific knowledge. It had taken a lifetime, since my pre-adolescence, to accumulate all my emotional and physical issues, and I couldn't expect to get rid of them overnight. I knew that I needed to practice patience and perseverance. It was not easy, but that's what I did. Months later I was already walking almost five miles a day, on my own and fast-paced. All my symptoms disappeared completely, except for a strong ringing in both ears due to the vertigo, but let's say I have learned to live with it. I joke and say, "What's a little buzzing for someone who couldn't even comb her own hair?" (laughs).

Definitely, I was born again. I once heard a patient who has been on the protocol longer than I have say that same thing – that he was born again after he met Dr. Cicero. He had no prospects of getting better, but then Dr. Cicero gave him his life back, all wrapped in a beautiful box with the words, "Here it is, go on and be happy."

And that is exactly the feeling I have now, I've received my life back, gift-wrapped. Year after year, the imaging tests confirm that I have made the best possible decision. Many lesions simply disappeared, others are still there, like scars, but there's been no progression of the disease. Absolutely no progression at all! This fact in itself is already cause for celebration, and my most profound gratitude to this doctor who has dedicated his life to his patients.

Today when I compare my reality to that of other patients who criticized me so much when I opted for an innovative way (yes, I faced a lot of criticism when I chose to start the Coimbra Protocol), sadness invades my heart. Many of them are already in wheelchairs; some can't see well, others are suffering from the prescription drugs' serious side effects, including PML. For me it's devastating to know that this is happening when there is a better option. I know very well how terrifying life is when you're going through a new relapse, waiting for steroid sessions in hospitals, and fearing an uncertain and painful future. And it's this feeling of nonconformity for something that can be easily changed with information which drives me to dedicate part of my time to take the good news to as many places as I can reach, through my experience.

Many other patients feel the same need to say how well and healthy they are. Relatives and friends of these patients also want to make their contribution. We are a group of people, from all over the world, who simply feel a moral duty to pass on information about what we have received. We want to share with others that, yes, there is a solution to autoimmune diseases. There is a solution to so much suffering and pain. I am a new person today. I think it is simply impossible to go through such a life experience – receiving the diagnosis of a progressive and incurable neurological disease, and right away finding a treatment that simply "switches off" this disease forever – and not to wake up from a deep sleep.

I feel that I was profoundly asleep. It's like I was with a blindfold that kept me from seeing nuances of my own personality; seeing traits that led me to self-boycott and to repeat patterns of behavior that betrayed me along the years. Finally, I could understand that our emotions have a major impact in every cell of our body. I still watch myself, and try not to overreact when facing the difficulties of everyday life. I try to be more indulgent with myself and less judgmental in life. I try not to let myself reach the stress levels I used to before, but if that happens, I know how to backtrack from it. I just let the river of life follows its course and then I go back to my balancing point. And that interview with Dr. Cicero on YouTube never left my mind: He said, "People in constant distress, people that are nervous and worry too much are more likely to develop neurodegenerative diseases."

To conclude my testimony, I must point out that ever since the world began, life revolves around the sun. How, then, have we come to think that we can just ignore this, and completely avoid the sun with impunity? How can we do without a mechanism that nature took millions of years to develop, in order to provide life on Earth, and simply not suffer the consequences? So let's wake up. Let's wake up from the deep sleep that modern life has brought with it and let's toast to the sun. Let's toast to life and its infinite possibilities. To vitamin D and the breaking of old paradigms.

Resources

Videos – Documentaries, Presentations and Interviews with Dr. Coimbra (English Subtitles)

Vitamina D – Por Uma Outra Terapia (English and Spanish subtitles) https://www.youtube.com/watch?v=erAgu1XcY-U

Coimbra, Vitamina D e Patologie Autoimmuni (English and Italian subtitles) https://www.youtube.com/watch?v=hOfO29rL-gI

Dr. Coimbra Explains his Treatment with High-Dose Vitamin D for Multiple Sclerosis (English subtitles – this was a presentation at the House Chamber of Representatives, in Brasilia, Federal Capital of Brazil.) https://www.youtube.com/watch?v=soK-M6z1cdiM

Dr. Michael Holick with Dr. Cicero Coimbra, in Brazil (Dr. Holick speaks in English, right at the beginning of the video.) https://www.youtube.com/watch?v=Cs5OXqyd8bk

Facebook Groups

Esclerose Múltipla – O Tratamento (Brazil) https://www.facebook.com/groups/EscleroseMultiplaOTratamento/

Per un'altra terapia – Vitamina D per la SM e per le malattie autoimmuni (Italy) https://www.facebook.com/groups/protocolloCoimbra/

Esclerosis Múltiple – Vitamina D – Latinoamerica (South America and Spain) https://www.facebook.com/groups/emperu/?fref=nf

Websites, Blogs and Forums

Vitamin D and Multiple Sclerosis http://www.vitamindandms.org/researchers/coimbra/index.html

MS Cure http://mscure.aussieblogs.com.au/the-bloggers-treatment-3/

Treating Multiple Sclerosis with high doses of vitamin D under medical supervision https://mscurevitamind.wordpress.com/

English information about Dr. Coimbra's treatment of MS with vitamin D (this is an Italian blog with an English section) https://vitaminadperlasclerosimultipla.wordpress.com/category/english-informations-about-dr-coimbras-treatment-of-ms-with-vitamin-d/

High Dosing vitD The Coimbra Protocol http://www.thisisms.com/forum/coimbra-high-dose-vitamin-d-protocol-f57/topic27020-15.html

Video Testimonies

Vitamina D Medicina e Saúde – Subtitled Videos (English)
http://www.vitaminadmedicinaesaude.com.br/category/subti-
tled-videos-english/
Esclerose Múltipla e Vitamina D (Multiple Sclerosis and High
Dose Vitamin D) – This is a video I made for the Vitamin D
Council Newsletter in Dec. 2014 (English)
https://www.youtube.com/watch?v=n4QyPA4SRQI

Updated List of Doctors

Google Maps: The Coimbra Protocol List of Doctors
https://www.google.com/maps/d/viewer?hl=en_US&app=mp&
mid=zK5He46-QQkM.kqPyJ2IosRyU

Endnotes

1 Cicero Galli Coimbra, MD, PHD, Department of Neurology and Neurosurgery, Federal University of São Paulo (UNIFESP), Laboratory of Clinical and Experimental Pathophysiology. (See Dr. Coimbra's Curriculum Vitae in Appendix.)

2 Ginde, Adit A; Liu, Mark C.; Camargo Carlos A. "Demographic Differences and Trends of Vitamin D Insufficiency in the US Population, 1988–2004." *Jama Internal Medicine* 169.6 (2009): 626-632.

3 IOM (Institute of Medicine). 2011. Dietary Reference Intakes for Calcium and Vitamin D. Washington, DC: The National Academies Press.

4 Smith, Philip. "Michael F. Holick, PhD, MD The Pioneer of Vitamin D Research." *Life Extension Magazine* Sep. 2010.

5 Passwater, Richard. "New Research on Vitamin D, Part 3: The Safety of Vitamin D. An Interview with John J. Cannell, M.D." *WholeFoods Magazine* Jul. 2011.

6 Nunes, Branca. "Cícero Galli Coimbra, o médico que trata a esclerose múltipla sem remédio." *Veja*, 25 Jun. 2014.

7 Burton, Jodie. "Is Vitamin D a Ray of Hope for Patients With MS?" *Neurology Reviews* 7;17.7 (2009) 1-16.

8 Laino, Charlene. "High Doses of Vitamin D Cut MS Relapses." *WebMD Health News*. 28 Apr. 2009. Retrieved from http://www.webmd.com/multiple-sclerosis/news/20090428/high-doses-vitamin-d-cut-ms-relapses.

9 Mok, Chi Chiu, Birmingham, Daniel, Rovin, Brad H.; Vitamin D Deficiency As Marker for Disease Activity and Organ Damage in Systemic Lupus Erythematosus: A Comparison with Anti-dsDNA and Anti-C1q. [abstract]. *Arthritis Rheum* 2011;63 Suppl 10 :2276.

10 Finamor, Danilo C; Coimbra, Rita Sinigaglia; Neves, Luiz C. M.; Gutierrez, Marcia; Silva, Jeferson J.;m Torres, Lucas D.; Surano, Fernanda; Neto, Domingos J.; Novo, Neil F.; Juliano, Yara; Lopes, Antonio C.; Coimbra, Cicero Galli. "A pilot study assessing the effect of prolonged administration of high daily doses of vitamin D on the clinical course of vitiligo and psoriasis." *Dermato-Endocrinology* 5.1 (2013): 222–234.

11 Mokry, Lauren E.; Ross, Stephanie; Ahmad, Omar S.; Forgetta, Vincenzo; Smith, George D.; Leong, Aaron; Greenwood, Celia M. T.; Thanassoulis, George; Richards, J. Brent. "Vitamin D and Risk of Multiple Sclerosis: A Mendelian Randomization Study." *PLOS Journal*, 25 Aug. 2015. DOI: 10.1371/journal.pmed.1001866.

12 Wahls, Terry. *The Wahls Protocol*. New York, NY: Avery, 2014. Print.

13 Mowry, E. M; Pelletier, D; Gao, Z; Howell, M. D; Zamvil, S. S; Waubant, E. "Vitamin D in clinically isolated syndrome: evidence for possible neuroprotection." *European Journal of Neurology*, 31 Oct. 2015. DOI: 10.1111/ene.12844.

14 Wright, Jonathan. *Why stomach acid is good for you*. New York, NY: M. Evans, 2001. Print.

15 Nouri, Mehrnaz; Bredberg, Anders; Weström, Björn; Lavasani, Shahram. "Intestinal Barrier Dysfunction Develops at the Onset of Experimental Autoimmune Encephalomyelitis, and Can Be Induced

by Adoptive Transfer of Auto-Reactive T Cells." *PLOS One*, Sep. 2014. DOI: 10.1371/journal.pone.0106335.

16 Wright, Jonathan; Lenard, Lane; (2001). *How Low Stomach Acid Can Make You Sick: The Bacteria-Cancer Connection. Why Stomach Acid Is Good For You* (pp. 121). New York, NY: M. Evans.

17 Boggild, Mike; Palace, Jack; Barton, Pelham; Ben-Shlomo, Yoav; Bregenzer, Thomas; Dobson, Charles; Gray, Richard. "Multiple sclerosis risk sharing scheme: two year results of clinical cohort study with historical comparator." *BMJ*. 2009; 339:b4677.

Ebers, G; Traboulsee, A; Li, D; et al. "Analysis of clinical outcomes according to original treatment groups 16 years after the pivotal IFNB-1b trial." *Journal of Neurology, Neurosurgery, and Psychiatry* 81.8 (2010): 907-12.

Veugelers, PJ; Fisk, JD; Brown, MG; Stadnyk, K; Sketris, IS; Murray, TJ; Bhan, V. "Disease progression among multiple sclerosis patients before and during a disease-modifying drug program: a longitudinal population-based evaluation." *Multiple Sclerosis* 15.11 (2009): 1286-94.

18 Boggild, Mike; Palace, Jack; Barton, Pelham; Ben-Shlomo, Yoav; Bregenzer, Thomas; Dobson, Charles; Gray, Richard. "Multiple sclerosis risk sharing scheme: two year results of clinical cohort study with historical comparator." *BMJ*. 2009; 339:b4677.

19 Woods, Alissa. "A Step Toward Multiple Sclerosis Treatment? Phase 2 ANTI-LINGO-1 Results Announced." *Multiple Sclerosis News Today*. 13 Jan. 2015. Retrieved from http://multiplesclerosisnewstoday.com/2015/01/13/a-step-toward-multiple-sclerosis-treatment-phase-2-anti-lingo-1-results-announced/.

20 Franklin, Robin; Kohlhaas, Susan. "Vitamin D could repair nerve damage in multiple sclerosis, study suggests." University of Cambridge. 07 Dec. 2015. Retrieved from https://www.cam.ac.uk/research/news/vitamin-d-could-repair-nerve-damage-in-multiple-sclerosis-study-suggests.

21 Cunha, Daniel. "Vitamina D – Por Uma Outra Terapia." Online Video. Youtube. Youtube, 11 April 2012. Web 18 December 2015.

Appendix

Cicero Galli Coimbra, MD, PHD
Department of Neurology and Neurosurgery
Federal University of São Paulo (UNIFESP)
Laboratory of Clinical and Experimental Pathophysiology

Academic Positions

2000-present
Associate Professor
Department of Neurology and Neurosurgery
Federal University of São Paulo (UNIFESP)
Laboratory of Clinical and Experimental Pathophysiology

1997-2000
Assistant Professor
Department of Neurology and Neurosurgery
Federal University of São Paulo (UNIFESP)
Laboratory of Clinical and Experimental Pathophysiology

1993-1997
Visiting Researcher
Department of Neurology and Neurosurgery
Federal University of São Paulo (UNIFESP)
Laboratory for Experimental Neurology

Activities

2010-present
Founder and President
Institute for Investigation and Treatment of Autoimmune Diseases

2006-present
Consultant Neurologist
Department of Medicine
Federal University of São Paulo (UNIFESP)

2003-present
Consultant Neurologist (Private Practice)

1998-present
Head of the Laboratory of Clinical and Experimental Pathophysiology
Department of Neurology and Neurosurgery
Federal University of São Paulo (UNIFESP)

1997-present
Assistant Professor
Department of Neurology and Neurosurgery
Federal University of São Paulo (UNIFESP)
Laboratory of Clinical and Experimental Pathophysiology

1990-2004
Preceptor and Attending Neurologist
Hospital of the Public Servant - São Paulo

1986-1988
Attending Neurologist
Hospital School at Federal University of São Paulo

Education

1999
Habilitation
Department of Neurology and Neurosurgery
Federal University of São Paulo (UNIFESP), Brazil

1991-1993
Post Doctorate
Laboratory for Experimental Brain Research
University of Lund, Sweden

1988-1991
Ph.D., Neurology
Laboratory for Experimental Neurology
Federal University of São Paulo (UNIFESP), Brazil

1986-1987
M.Sc., Neurology
Laboratory for Experimental Neurology
Federal University of São Paulo (UNIFESP), Brazil

1984-1985
Fellowship in Pediatric Neurology
Jackson Memorial Hospital in Miami, USA

1981-1982
Residency in Adult Neurology
Federal University of Rio Grande do Sul (UFRGS), Brazil

1979-1980
Residency in Internal Medicine

Federal University of Rio Grande do Sul (UFRGS), Brazil
1974-1979
Graduation in Medicine
Federal University of Rio Grande do Sul (UFRGS), Brazil

Awards and Honors

2008
Brazil's most admired medical doctors ("Análise Editorial" Magazine, Brazil)

2002
Poster Award - World Federation of Neurology
II International Congress on Vascular Dementia – Salzburg, Austria

1994
Autregésilo Research Award – National Academy of Medicine (Brazil)

Publications

Book Chapters

SINIGAGLIA-COIMBRA, R.; LOPES, Antonio Carlos; COIM-BRA, C. / COIMBRA, C.G. Chapter 153 - Riboflavin, brain function and health. Part 24 - Starvation and nutrient deficiency. In: Victor R Preedy; Ronald R Watson; Colin R Martin. (Org.). The International Handbook of Behavior, Diet and Nutrition. The International Handbook of Behavior, Diet and Nutrition. 1ed.London: Springer, 2011, v. 4, p. 2427-2449.

SINIGAGLIA-COIMBRA, Rita; BORGES, Andréa Aurélio; GRASSL, Christian; LOPES, Antonio Carlos ; COIMBRA, C. / COIMBRA, C.G. III. Hyperthermia following ischemia-reperfusion as a valuable tool for pre-clinical development of therapeutic strategies relevant to human dementias. In: Ryszard Pluta. (Org.). Ischemia-reperfusion pathways in Alzheimer's Disease. Ischemia-reperfusion pathways in Alzheimer's Disease. 1ed.Hauppauge: Nova Science Publishers, 2007, v. 1, p. -.

COIMBRA, C. / COIMBRA, C.G. Are brain dead (or brain-stem dead) patients neurologically recoverable?. In: Roberto Mattei. (Org.). Finis Vitae - Is brain death still life? Finis Vitae - Is brain death still life?. 2ed.Calábria: Rubbettino Editore, 2007, v. 1.

COIMBRA, C. / COIMBRA, C.G. The apnea test - A bedside lethal 'disaster' to avoid a legal 'disaster' in the operating room. In: Roberto de Mattei. (Org.). Finis Vitae - Is brain death still life?. Finis Vitae - Is brain death still life?. 1ed.Calábria: Rubbettino Editore, 2006, v. 1, p. 336-.

Articles

Favero-Filho, L.A.; Borges, A.A.; Grassl, C.; Lopes, A.C.; COIMBRA, C. / COIMBRA, C.G; Coimbra, C.G. Hyperthermia induced after recirculation triggers chronic neurodegeneration in the penumbra zone of focal ischemia in the rat brain. Brazilian Journal of Medical and Biological Research (Impresso) v. 41, p. 1029-1036, 2008.

DALPAI, Janise; BORGES, Andréa Aurélio; GRASSL, Christian; FAVEROFILHO, Luiz Antonio; XAVIER, Gilberto Fernando; JUNQUEIRA, Virginia Berlanga Camargo; LOPES, Antonio Carlos; COIMBRA, C. / COIMBRA, C.G; SINIGAGLIA-COIMBRA, Rita.

Dietary riboflavin restriction abd chronic hemin administration does not alter brain function in rats: The importance of vitamin homeostasis in the brain. Current Topics in Nutraceutical Research, v. 5, p. 101-108, 2007.

COIMBRA, C. / COIMBRA, C.G; JUNQUEIRA, Virginia Berlanga Camargo. Response to the Comments of H.B. Ferraz et al. about the paper "High doses of riboflavin and the elimination of dietary red meat promote the recovery of some motor functions in Parkinson's disease patients. Brazilian Journal of Medical and Biological Research, v. 37, p. 1297-1302, 2004.

COIMBRA, C. / COIMBRA, C.G; JUNQUEIRA, V. B. C. High doses of riboflavin and the elimination of dietary red meat significantly promote the recovery of some motor functions in Parkinson's disease. Brazilian Journal of Medical and Biological Research, v. 39, n.10, p. 1409-1417, 2003.

SINIGAGLIA-COIMBRA, R.; CAVALHEIRO, Esper Abrão; COIMBRA, C. / COIMBRA, C.G. Postischemic hyperthermia induces Alzheimer-like pathology in the rat brain. Acta Neuropathologica, Berlin, v. 103, n.5, p. 444-452, 2002.

SINIGAGLIA-COIMBRA, Rita; CAVALHEIRO, Esper Abrão; COIMBRA, C. / COIMBRA, C.G. Protective effect of systemic treatment with cylosporine A after global ischemia in rats. Journal of the Neurological Sciences, Amsterdam, v. 203-4, p. 273-276, 2002.

COIMBRA, C. / COIMBRA, C.G. Morte cerebral. Falhas nos critérios de diagnóstico. Ciência Hoje, Rio de Janeiro RJ, v. 27, n.161, p. 26-30, 2000.

COIMBRA, C. / COIMBRA, C.G. Implications of ischemic pemumbra for the diagnosis of brain death. Brazilian Journal of Medical and Biological Research, São Paulo, v. 32, n.12, p. 1479-1488, 1999.

COIMBRA, C. / COIMBRA, C.G. Morte encefálica: um diagnóstico agonizante. Revista de Neurociências, São Paulo, v. 6, n.2, p. 58-68, 1998.

COIMBRA, C. / COIMBRA, C.G; BORIS-MÖLLER, F.; DRAKE, M.; WIELOCH, T. Diminished neuronal damage in the rat brain by late treatment with the antipyretic dipyrone or cooling following cerebral ischemia. Acta Neuropathologica, v. 92, p. 447-453, 1996.

COIMBRA, C. / COIMBRA, C.G; DRAKE, M.; BORIS-MÖLLER, F.; WIELOCH, T. Long-lasting neuroprotective effect of postischemic hypothermia and treatment with an anti-inflammatory/antipyretic drug: evidence for chronic encephalopathic processes following ischemia. Stroke, v. 27, p. 1578-1585, 1996.

COIMBRA, C. / COIMBRA, C.G; CARVALHO, A C; OLIVEIRA, R. J.; SINIGAGLIA, R.; SANTOS, G.; CAVALHEIRO, Esper Abrão. Effects of reperfusion under moderate hypothermia on ischemic brain damage. Ciência e Cultura (SBPC), v. 47, p. 266-268, 1995.

CARVALHO, A C; OLIVEIRA, R. J.; SINIGAGLIA, R.; SANTOS, G.; COIMBRA, C. / COIMBRA, C.G; CAVALHEIRO, Esper Abrão. Efeitos da reperfuSão sob hipotermia moderada na lesão cerebral isquêmica. Ciência e Cultura (SBPC), São Paulo, v. 47, n.4, p. 266-268, 1995.

COIMBRA, C. / COIMBRA, C.G; WIELOCH, T. Moderate hypothermia mitigates neuronal damage in the rat brain when initiated several hours following transient cerebral ischemia. Acta Neuropathologica, v. 87, p. 325-331, 1994.

COIMBRA, C. / COIMBRA, C.G; WIELOCH, T. Hypothermia ameliorates neuronal survival when induced 2 hours after ischaemia in the rat. Acta Physiologica Scandinavica, v. 146, p. 543-544, 1992.

COIMBRA, C. / COIMBRA, C.G; CAVALHEIRO, Esper Abrão. Protective effect of short-term post-ischemic hypothermia on the gerbil brain. . Brazilian Journal of Medical and Biological Research, v. 23, p. 605-611, 1990.

COIMBRA, C. / COIMBRA, C.G; CIFUENTES, F. E.; CAVALHEIRO, Esper Abrão. Thyroid hormones and the pathophysiology of brain ischemia. Ciência e Cultura (SBPC), v. 42, p. 471-475, 1990.

COIMBRA, C. / COIMBRA, C.G; CIFUENTES, F. E.; CAVALHEIRO, Esper Abrão. Correlation of postural and pathological findings in a modified four vessel occlusion model of rat forebrain ischemia. Brazilian Journal of Medical and Biological Research, v. 22, p. 1237-1250, 1989.

TURSKI, W. A.; CAVALHEIRO, Esper Abrão; COIMBRA, C. / COIMBRA, C.G; BERZAGHI, M. P.; IKONOMIDOU-TURSKI, C.; TURSKI, L. Only certain antiepileptic drugs prevent seizures induced by pilocarpine. Brain Research, v. 434, p. 281-305, 1987.

Made in the USA
San Bernardino, CA
29 March 2019